CBD Hemp Oil

101

The Essential Beginner's Guide to Improve Your Health, Cure Diseases, Reduce Pain, and Anxiety

Joshua Grannus © 2018

Legal Disclaimer

CONTENTS

INTRODUCTION - A BRIEF HISTORY OF EVOLUTION 1

CHAPTER ONE – 16

EMERGENCE OF CBD OIL FROM HEMP OIL 16

WHAT IS HEMP? HOW IS IT DIFFERENT FROM CANNABIS/MARIHUANA? 16

HEMP OIL: WHAT IS IT AND WHERE DOES IT COME FROM? 18

HEMP SEED OIL DOSAGE: HOW MUCH IS TOO MUCH? 19

HEMP OIL BENEFITS: HOW GOOD IS IT FOR THE BODY? 21

HEMP OIL: POTENTIAL ADVERSE EFFECTS THROUGH MISUSE 23

CBD HEMP OIL/ CBD OIL: WHAT IS IT AND WHERE DOES IT COME FROM? .. 23

CBD HEMP OIL DOSAGE: HOW TO TAKE IT AS A SUPPLEMENT? 26

CBD HEMP OIL BENEFITS: HOW GOOD IS IT FOR MY BODY? 28

CBD HEMP OIL AND ITS SIDE EFFECTS THROUGH MISUSE 32

CHAPTER TWO - PHYSICAL BENEFITS OF CBD HEMP OIL 34

CBD HEMP OIL AS A BONE STIMULANT 35

Osteoporosis 36

Osteoarthritis 37

Rheumatoid arthritis (RA): 38

USE OF CDB HEMP OIL FOR BONE DISORDER AND DISEASES 38

CBD HEMP OIL AS ANTI-BACTERIAL AND ANTI-PSORIATIC 39

Acne 40

Eczema 41

Psoriasis 42

Skin Wounds 43

Scalp Care 44

USE OF CDB HEMP OIL FOR SKIN CONDITIONS AND WOUNDS 45

CBD HEMP OIL AS AN IMMUNOSUPPRESSIVE 46

Multiple Sclerosis 48

Lupus 49

Cancer 50

USE OF CDB HEMP OIL FOR AUTOIMMUNE DISEASES 52

CBD HEMP OIL AS AN ANTI-DIABETIC 54

Type 1 Diabetes..55

Type 2 Diabetes...57

Obesity 59

Diabetic Retinopathy..60

USE OF CDB HEMP OIL FOR DIABETIC DISEASES..............................61

CBD HEMP OIL AS AN ANALGESIC...62

Chronic Pain...63

Back Pain 66

Fibromyalgia 67

Migraines...69

Menstrual Cramps..70

USE OF CDB HEMP OIL FOR CHRONIC PAIN AND RELATED ISSUES 71

CBD HEMP OIL AS INTESTINAL ANTI-PROKINETIC AND APPETITE STIMULANT ...74

Gastritis 76

Peptic Ulcers and Gastric Ulcers 78

Crohn's Disease...81

Eating Disorders..84

USE OF CDB HEMP OIL FOR DIGESTIVE AND INFLAMMATORY DISEASES 86

CBD HEMP OIL AS ANTI-EPILEPTIC AND ANTI-SPASMODIC......................90

MUSCLE SPASMS 93

EPILEPSY 95

LENNOX-GASTAUT/DRAVIT/WEST SYNDROME 98

USE OF CDB HEMP OIL FOR SEIZURE AND SPASTIC DISORDERS..................99

CBD HEMP OIL AN ANTI-ISCHEMIC 102

CARDIOVASCULAR DISEASES 105

CONGENITAL HEART DEFECT..110

USE OF CDB HEMP OIL FOR HEART DISEASES..................................114

CBD HEMP OIL AS AN ANTIFUNGAL 116

ATHLETE'S FOOT/ RINGWORM/ JOCK ITCH.....................................119

YEAST INFECTION 120

USE OF CBD HEMP OIL FOR FUNGAL INFECTIONS 122

CHAPTER FOUR - PSYCHOLOGICAL BENEFITS OF CBD HEMP OIL 125

CBD HEMP OIL AS ANTI-ANXIOLYTIC 128

ANXIETY DISORDERS 131

DEPRESSION 133

ANXIETY AND PANIC ATTACKS 136

SUBSTANCE ABUSE AND DEPENDENCY DISORDER 141

USE OF CBD HEMP OIL FOR ANXIETY DISORDERS 145

CBD HEMP OIL AS AN ANTIPSYCHOTIC 148

SCHIZOPHRENIA 152

BIPOLAR PSYCHOSIS 155

SUBSTANCE-INDUCED PSYCHOSIS 157

USE OF CBD HEMP OIL AS AN ANTIPSYCHOTIC 160

CHAPTER FIVE - CBD STRAINS AND EXTRACTS 166

TYPES OF EXTRACT 167

HIGH-CBD OIL 168

CBD HEMP OIL 169

TYPES OF STRAINS 170

CHARLOTTE'S WEB 170

ACDC 172

CANNA-TSU 173

SOUR TSUNAMI 175

CANNATONIC 177

HARLEQUIN 179

HARLE-TSU 181

RINGO'S GIFT 183

ONE TO ONE 185

CBD CRITICAL CURE 187

CALI CURE 189

DESERT RUBY 190

REMEDY 192

DANCEHALL 193

SUZY Q 195

DANCE WORLD 197

CBD SHARK 198

PENNYWISE 199

CORAZÓN 201

VALENTINE X 203

SPECIFIED STRAINS FOR VARIOUS DISORDERS 205

PRECAUTIONS FOR USING STRAINS 215

CHAPTER SIX - A BRIEF GUIDE TO A HEALTHIER LIFE **218**

JUMP ON TO THE NUTRITION BANDWAGON 218

INTAKE OF IRON 219

INTAKE OF PROTEIN 220

INTAKE OF HEALTHIER FATS AND OILS 221

HEALTHIER INGREDIENT CHOICES 222

THE 5-A-DAY RULE 227

FOLLOW A SET EXERCISE ROUTINE 229

INCORPORATING SUPPLEMENTS WITH THE WORKOUT 229

SIMPLE HOME WORKOUTS 230

RELAX YOUR MIND 232

FIND A CALMER STATE OF MIND 233

CHAPTER SEVEN - HEALTHY CBD HEMP OIL/ HEMP OIL/ HEMP SEED RECIPES. **235**

VEGAN HEMP SEED PESTO 236

    Ingredients *236*

    Direction *237*

RAW FOOD TRAIL MIX 237

    Ingredients *238*

    Directions *239*

SUPERFOOD SALAD 240

    Ingredients *240*

    Directions *241*

TABOULI SALAD 243

    Ingredients *243*

    Directions *244*

HEMP AND CARROT SOUP 244

    Ingredients *244*

    Directions *245*

SPICY CHICKPEAS AND CUCUMBER SALAD 246

    Ingredients *246*

    Directions *247*

HEMP BURGERS 248

    Ingredients *248*

Directions...249

TOFU TACOS...249

Ingredients...249

Directions...250

GRILLED TOMATO SALSA 251

Ingredients...251

Directions...252

VEGAN MAC N CHEESE 252

Ingredients...252

Directions...253

CREAMY AVOCADO PASTA...254

Ingredients...255

Directions...255

VEGAN CHILLI 256

Ingredients...256

Directions...257

PEANUT BUTTER GRANOLA...258

Ingredients...258

Directions...258

HIDDEN GREEN POWER SMOOTHIE 259

Ingredients...259

Directions...260

GREEN WARRIOR PROTEIN SMOOTHIE.........................260

Ingredients...260

Directions...261

FRUIT KABOBS..261

Ingredients...262

Directions...263

CHOCOLATE ALMOND FROZEN BANANA POPS 263

Ingredients...263

Directions...264

BANANA CREAM PIE BLIZZARDS................................265

Ingredients...265

Directions...266

CONCLUSION **267**

REFERENCES..270

INTRODUCTION - A BRIEF HISTORY OF EVOLUTION

Along with the passage of history, hemp or its constituents has been considered one of the most valuable discoveries due to its competent and multi-usage capabilities. In the modern day and age, not much is known about hemp other than it being used as a medicinal drug or recreational one.

However, it has been serving people of the past in many fields as an ideal plant, kind of like the jack of all trades. The very first instances of cultivating hemp were found 10,000 years ago, where it served as a soil conditioner due to its replenishing properties. It served as a fertilizer that would revitalize the soil while adding nutrients, oxygen, and nitrogen into the ground. This benefited the farmers by allowing them to easily rotate crops such as legumes and corn into the plots.

Not only did it create a healthy soil environment for other crops, but it also helped them grow a stronger root system. The hemp plant can grow up to 10 to 20 feet tall, while its root system develops in a mesh-like pattern that could support other plant roots in soil that has been compromised due to flooding. The benefits of the hemp plant do not stop here, other parts of the plant were actively used due to its durability.

For example, the fiber of this plant is very strong; it is one of the naturally occurring fibers in the world. Moreover, the ratio of fiber produced through the hemp plant and the pine tree is 4:1. The hemp fiber was also found to be used for equipment and tools in 8000 B.C.

After 2000 years, it had found an active place in the Ancient Chinese market. They used it as a building material and for shoes and clothing. Conversely, the ancient Chinese civilization had also discovered the medicinal properties of this plant, categorizing it as a herb. They found out that its seed was jam-packed with vitamin, protein, amino acids, and essential fatty acids. The medicinal properties of the hemp plant grew its popularity in the area, and its other parts like the stalk and its seed were used to make salves and hemp oil.

To put it another way, the hemp plant had been known for its health benefits before its rise of popularity in the western societies. The Ancient Chinese civilization also used the hemp fruit as food due to it calming properties, which lead to the research of it as medicine.

Through the research of the oldest pharmacopeia in Chinese literature known as the *"PenTs'ao Ching"* or translated as *"The Herbal"*, the hemp plant was categorized as dioecious. In this book, the hemp plant was recognized to be either female or male.

Whereas, the counterparts of the hemp plant complimented each other, spiritually and physically. This idea was taken from the philosophy of Yin and Yang from the Taoist religion. This Daoism emphasized the harmony of the twin nature of this plant, giving it a wizardly appeal of transcendentalism and spiritual immortality. See, the nature of yin and yang had built an ongoing appeal to this plant as a method to achieve tranquility and peace to reach a spontaneous and harmonious existence. Surprisingly, this duality still exists in the clinical world and was differentiated by their common identities; namely, marijuana and industrial hemp.

Going back to the historical simile of Yin and Yang, the hemp plant had achieved its dual nature due to the female and male counterpart. The female hemp plant, if allowed to grow completely, produced flowers that would offer "shelter" to the wandering and lost spirits, connecting it to Yin. While, the male plant that does not grow a flower when matured is considered as the yang, the stronger counterpart.

In the Ancient Chinese civilization, it was found that while the experimentation of the female and the male plant had been occurring, there was no written evidence about the fact. The first recorded use of hemp as a medicinal herb in history was found to be in *"PenTs'ao Ching,"* which referred to it as a spiritual and mystic plant that could be used in teas. Moreover, the Emperor Shen-Nung referenced it directly because of his active use of this plant due to its medicinal properties. You would think, living in the past ages and not having information on the proper effects of an herb would have stopped Shen-Nung from further research on the hemp plant.

However, it only further instigated him to research other effects of the plant. It was initially used as a laxative that offered relief for intestinal issues; this was essential because the seeds contained proteins and fatty acids. Through modern research, it has been found the existence of fatty acids like g-linoleic acid that have therapeutic effects that could provide relief for intestinal issues. The textual evidence has pointed to the fact that Shen-Nung used hemp by extracting its oil by pressing the seeds. He used the oils to make herbal teas that were described to help natural pains and give quick relief.

It must also be noted; on the discovery of its medicinal properties, the hemp plant has also experimented for its other uses. Shen-Nung used the hemp seed residue left to create a balm-like ointment that is to be considered as the first topical hemp item made in history. This balm was used to treat skin irritation and rashes; the texts also suggest it was being used to treat the symptoms of intestinal constipation, disruption of the female reproductive system, malaria, rheumatic pain, and many other similar issues.

Another key point of its popularity or decline of one was due to it being referenced as a psychoactive drug in the *Pen-ts'aoching*. The association of hemp and its hallucinogenic properties were mentioned in this book due to it being used in shamanism by the residents of Central Asia.

During the Han dynasty, such religious practices became a reason for disbelief; they were increasingly forgotten due to the heavy restrictions placed by the government. The gradual decrease in the usage in China brought the dissemination of the properties of hemp plant to Western Asia and India.

Following this time, around 1000 B.C., the Hemp industry boomed in India and maintained its strong connection with medicine and spiritualism. The experimentation of the hemp plant in this region produced three different types of hemp forms; named from the weakest to strongest as Bhang, Ganja, and Charas. Spiritually, the hemp plant was mentioned in the sacred text known as *Atharva Veda* to be as five sacred plants merged in one to bring happiness, joy, relief, and freedom.

It was used medicinally for its various functions and uses; it was used as an analgesic for a headache, toothache, and neuralgia, it was used as an anticonvulsant to treat rabies and tetanus, it was used as tranquilizer and hypnotic to treat mania, anxiety, and hysteria, it was used as an anti-inflammatory to find for inflammatory diseases, it was used as an antibiotic through topical usage on erysipelas, skin infections, and tuberculosis, it was used as an anti-parasite drug to treat internal and external worms, it was used as an antispasmodic for diarrhea and colic disease. Other uses of hemp in the Indian history were as an antitussive, expectorant, appetite stimulant, diuretic, and a digestive herb.

The hemp plant's population delved very deep in southern Asia, from where it spread to the Middle Eastern areas and Africa. During the 1000 A.D., it was noted through textual evidence that Muslim used it as herbal medicine. It commonly used to 'clean the brain' and as a digestive, diuretic, and anti-flatulent herbal remedy. (1) It was used as a remedial and healing plan in the African regions, notably to facilitate childbirth, fever, malaria, snake bite, asthma, dysentery, and anthrax. (2) Initially, the use of hemp for the treatment of various ailments was brought in South America by the African slaves. It was used synonymously by the Blacks that were residents of the Angola region, particularly, the northeastern rural areas. It has been reportedly used in these rural areas for the treatment of menstrual cramps and toothache. (2) During this time, the production of the hemp plant was introduced in Europe through the cultivation of its stem fiber.

Around 1150, the description of the hemp plant is found in many books; it was described as an herbal remedy to various issues. However, it was not until the 18th century that the distinction of the male and female hemp plant was found, other than that of the Chinese simile of Yin and Yang.

It is important to realize that it was not until the mid of 19th century that the western medical community began the research of this mystical plant that had been used as a remedy for many and all kinds of ailments. Through the research of Willian B. O'Shaughnessy and Jacques-Joseph Moreau, the proper effects of the hemp plant were found out. O'Shaughnessy was French physician that worked for the British in India, where he first came in contact with a strand of the hemp extract. He researched on its effects and read popular literature on this nature and characteristics of this plant. He tested the effects of this plant on animals and later, it was clinically tested on patients with various pathologies. He published 'O*n the preparations of the Indian hemp, or gunjah*' in 1939, in which he described the uses of the plant as:

"The narcotic effects of Hemp are popularly known in the south of Africa, South America, Turkey, Egypt, Middle East Asia, India, and the adjacent territories of the Malays, Burmese, and Siamese. In all these countries, Hemp is used in various forms, by the dissipated and depraved, as the ready agent of a pleasing intoxication. In the popular medicine of these nations, we find it extensively employed for a multitude of affections. But in Western Europe, its use either as a stimulant or as a remedy is equally unknown" (3)

Later in his work, he extensively describes the successful treatment of convulsions, rheumatism, and muscular spasms through various form of hemp extract. This, solidly, laid rest to many uncertainties about the nature of this plant such as it is a mystical or blessed plant that had religious connotations.

Moreau, on the other hand, had different plans of research for this particular plant. He worked as an assistant physician for the Charenton Asylum. During that time, it was common practice for a therapist to accompany patients during their long trips to distant lands. On one of his visits to Arab, he noticed that Hashish (hemp resin) was being used to various maladies. This peaked his curiosity and led him to experiment with the different kinds Hemp seed raisin and oils on himself and his assistants.

Accordingly, after the experiment, he found many acute effects of different preparation of hemp seed and raisin. In 1845 he published a book named *'Du Hachischet de l'AlienationMentale: Etudes Psychologiques,'* in which he clearly stated that it was a powerful therapeutic remedy for mental illnesses. He says that: "...I saw in hashish, more specifically in its effects on mental abilities, a powerful and unique method to investigate the genesis of mental illness". (4)

For this reason, the research on hemp plant and its various forms, particularly for its therapeutic and psychoactive effects have persisted over the course of years. The western medicinal world, through the contribution of O'Shaughnessy and Moreau, has been significantly impacted. The scarcity of a treatment option for tetanus, cholera, and rabies has also been one of the reasons for its popularity. The use of this plant as a topical, herbal, therapeutic, and psychotic medicine spread from China to Indian, from India to the Eastern areas, which quickly grabbed the interest of French and European men of medicine. The first ever clinical conference about the nature of Hemp was held in 1860, it was organized in America by the Ohio State Medical Society.

By the end of the 19th century, more than 100 clinical and scientific articles had been published that described in detail the medical value and effect of the hemp plant. Inevitably, it boomed in popularity and was largely marketed as tinctures or extracts of a different part of the Hemp plant.

In 1924, The Analytic Cyclopedia of Practical Medicine described and summarized all of the medical uses and effects of Hemp by categorizing it in three areas. It acted as a hypnotic and sedative for senile insomnia, chorea, melancholia, pulmonary tuberculosis, insomnia, delirium tremens, spasm of the bladder, gonorrhea, hay fever, and bronchitis. It acted as an analgesic that brought relief during migraines, headache, brain tumors, multiple neuritis, eye-strain, postpartum hemorrhage, menorrhagia, dental pain, gastralgia (indigestion), uterine disturbances, tingling, numbness of gout, eczema, brain tumors, neuralgia, tic douloureux, and acute rheumatism. Lastly, it was categorized as an herbal remedy for digestion and appetite issues, anorexia, neurosis, diarrhea, cholera, dyspepsia, palpitation, vertigo, diabetes mellitus, hematuria, nephritis, impotence males and sexual atony in females.

As with all prevalent peculiarities in the world, the beginning of the 20th century brought a decline in the use of hemp or as its popular counterpart marijuana both of which are a classification of the same species Cannabis Sativa. During this time, the better parts of the plant had been distinguished; they were commonly used in the form of crude extracts and tinctures whose value depended upon the mode of preparation, origin, and age.

Following the implication, many legal restrictions, such as the Marihuana Tax Act, were placed that restricted the use and growth of this plant. Due to the excessive paperwork following the taxation and fine for the purpose of the plant, the Supreme Court gave the States control over the transaction, which ultimately led to banning of the plant as a whole. It was removed from the official pharmacopeia of America in 1941.

The second half of the 20th century brought this plant closer to the social world of literature; it was consumed for hedonistic purposes in many instances. Intellectuals from all over the world used it to bloom their imagination in gatherings or in the tranquility of their rooms to get inspiration for their works.

The recreational use of hemp and its derivatives had reached one of the highest points in history, where it was used by young adults 64% of the times in 1982. (5) During this explosion of importance, the scientific research grew fond of researching the hemp plant. In 1964, this research led to the discovery of the chemical structure of D9-THC, which was one of the active constituents of the plant. Mecholuam brought this prolific contribution to the medical world.

Later, a study by the International Association of Plant Taxonomy in 1976 concluded that: "both hemp varieties and marijuana varieties are of the same genus, Cannabis, and the same species, Cannabis Sativa. Further, countless varieties fall into further classifications within the species Cannabis Sativa." Where the growth and breeding of the plant determined its classification as either marijuana/cannabis or hemp.

This scientific interest brought many discoveries that brought accurate therapeutic effects of the hemp plant where D9-THC, in particular, was used to treat conditions such as spams, vomiting, insomnia, and so forth. Many other cannabinoids were found as the constituents of the hemp plant, which exhibited different effects for different ailments. Cannabidiol (CBD) was one of the major constituents of the hemp plant that was proven as an analgesic, anti-emetic, stimulant of appetite, and treatment for Multiple Sclerosis. (6) With the intention to heal and contribute to the medical world multinational pharmaceutical laboratory was granted approval to market medication with constituents of the hemp plant, provided that they contained CBD or D9-THC for relief. It started a new cycle of derivatives of the hemp plant that consisted of compounds with different marked effectiveness. The treatment through this endogenous cannabinoid system of remedies was finally scientifically proven and safely procured by companies all over the world.

CHAPTER ONE – EMERGENCE OF CBD OIL FROM HEMP OIL

WHAT IS HEMP? HOW IS IT DIFFERENT FROM CANNABIS/MARIHUANA?

Hemp is a species of the Cannabaceae family, which is grown in a natural environment by sowing the Cannabis Sativa plant. This species of the Cannabaceae family naturally grows in the northern areas. It grows tall with sturdy stem structure and long leaves. The height of a fully grown hemp plant can range up to 20 feet, or longer in varied species. The period of growth and maturation for this particular plant can range from ten to sixteen weeks. Due to the lack of education and social stigma surrounding the Cannabaceae family, one may be forced to ask at this point to be clarified about hemp and its popular counterpart known as cannabis or marijuana.

Cannabis or Marijuana is differentiated by the breeding of the Cannabis Sativa plant. If the Cannabis

Sativa plant is grown and bred for the resinous glands that have potent psychoactive properties, then it would be described as cannabis. The psychoactive property comes from the high levels of tetrahydrocannabinol (THC) in the trichomes (the glands). Tetrahydrocannabinol (THC) is a popular constituent of the Sativa plant, which is produced when the naturally present Cannabigerolic acid (CBGA) in the plant is exposed to UV light and heat. The Cannabigerolic acid (CBGA) is a precursor to other cannabinoids such as Cannabidiol (CBD), Tetrahydrocannabinol (THC), and Cannabichromene (CBC).

Hemp or Industrial hemp, alternatively, is identified in as Cannabis Sativa plant that produces low traces of Tetrahydrocannabinol (THC). This plant is harvested for industrial use; it typically has been grown to make topical ointments, oils, and other times for construction and clothing. The legal levels of THC that could be present in the Sativa plant are less than 0.3%. This single factor contributes to the differentiation of what is classified as hemp or cannabis/marijuana.

HEMP OIL: WHAT IS IT AND WHERE DOES IT COME FROM?

Hemp Oil or Hempseed Oil is derived from hemp seeds that are cold pressed to get unrefined oil. It has a light color that is clear and has a taste of nuttiness. This oil is made explicitly by pressing the seeds of industrial hemp seeds, not the Sativa flowers containing high levels of THC. This oil is primarily used in body care products because of its high nutritional value; it contains omega-6 and omega-3 essential fatty acids. The seed of naturally occurring Sativa plant does not contain any THC. Thus it does not have any cannabinoids. For this reason, industrial hemp oil is commonly used in paints, inks, lubricants plastics. It is also added to shampoos and detergents.

Going father to dig out its nutrient content, it has some essential fatty acids(EFAs) such as omega -6, linoleic, omega-3, alpha-linolenic acid, stearidonic acid, and gamma-linolenic acid. Taking one tablespoon of hempseed oil would provide the daily requirement of EFA for humans. It has also been noted that the continuous use of hemp oil will not cause an imbalance of essential fatty acids, unlike flaxseed oil.

HEMP SEED OIL DOSAGE: HOW MUCH IS TOO MUCH?

Hemp oil has a grassy aroma that has a distinct aftertaste, which can only be found if it is cold pressed. The seed oil of an industrial hemp plan has a very low cannabinoid percentage. Furthermore, it is processed later on to remove any cannabinoid content to heighten the nutrition value. The oil contains thirty to thirty-five percent of nutritious oil content that includes eighty percent essential fatty acids. As mentioned above; it has a 55% of omega-6 and linoleic acid, 22% of omega-3 and alpha-linolenic acid, 4 % of omega-6 and gamma-linolenic acid, and 2% of stearidonic acid.

The ratio of the unsaturated fat and saturated fat percentage in hemp seed oil is three to one. The saturated fats are known to raise the cholesterol levels while increasing the chance of 2 type diabetes and heartache. However, it is found in many common foods such as red meat, chicken products, dairies such as cheese, shortening, and butter. On the other hand, Unsaturated fats are healthier than the alternative.

They are commonly found in nuts, seeds, and vegetables. The unsaturated fats have two kinds known as monounsaturated fats and polyunsaturated fats. The monounsaturated fats can improve cholesterol levels and lessen the risk of cardiovascular disease. The polyunsaturated fats are divided into Omega-3 fatty acids and Omega-6 fatty acids. The recommended dosage of omega-3to get maximum health benefits by the European Food Safety Authority is 2.25 grams. Whereas, the recommended dosage of omega-6 is 6 to 10 grams daily. The recommended fat intake by the American Heart Association 25% to 35%, where the saturated content should be lower than 7% of your daily calorie diet.

A point to take notice is that the ratio of the perfect and healthiest dosage of omega-3 to omega-6 for humans is 3:1. While every hundred grams of hemp oil has 55 to 60 percent omega-6 and 22 to 23 percent omega-3 fatty acids. The optimal dosage through this estimate could be counted as approximately sixteen grams of hemp oil daily. To put it in simpler words, one tablespoon of hemp oil could contribute to a healthier body and spirit. Taking two or more than two tablespoons would excessive and may cause adverse effects.

HEMP OIL BENEFITS: HOW GOOD IS IT FOR THE BODY?

Hemp oil has been profoundly favorite in the vegan community because of its nutritional value. It has a high content of the right fatty acids that help improve the health. It contains those fatty acids that the body does not produce on its own; these are not always perfectly proportioned in most of the foods in the everyday lifestyle. It has polyunsaturated fats such as Omega-3 and Omega-6 that help individuals find themselves in better health conditions.

Omega-3 has been known to optimize the lipid production and profile that further lessens the chance of chronic cardiovascular disease. Research has also shown that regular digestion of omega-3 had drastically lowered the chances of cardiac-related diseases. Omega-6 acids, on the other hand, help the nervous system maintain an optimal condition, it also plays an essential role in repairing damaged tissues.

Hemp oil has been used for ages as a vitamin supplement; it has been used to treat countless ailments. It helps the circulatory system and maintains a healthy environment that prevents it from developing heart conditions such as hypotension and hypertension. It also helps calm down the irritated skin areas.

Moreover, it can also treat acne and eczema. It helps maintain a healthy body that could aid treatment for diabetes. The immune system of the body is also given a boost through the regular use of hemp oil; this could keep minor illnesses such as flu or cold away. Hormone imbalance is also maintained through the frequent use of hemp oil; it could lower the PMS and menstrual cramp symptoms. Moreover, it could also be used as an alternative to other saturated fatty oils in foods to prepare nutritious and healthier meals.

HEMP OIL: POTENTIAL ADVERSE EFFECTS THROUGH MISUSE

Hempseed oil has been known to have many beneficial qualities that could help maintain a healthier body through regular and optimum usage. However, if it is used in excess, it could cause an adverse side effect, albeit, very mild. Some studies have shown that the use of hemp orally or topically has some mild side effects that could cause low blood pressure, lightheadedness, and dryness of mouth.

The toxicity of hemp was studied after this concern; however, even after taking the dose up to 300 times, there was no toxic threat level found. Conversely, hempseed oil is considered to be an anticoagulant, which is why it is recommended to be used with caution by people with hemophilia.

CBD HEMP OIL/ CBD OIL: WHAT IS IT AND WHERE DOES IT COME FROM?

Cannabidiol (CBD) Hemp Oil is produced from the seed and stalk of a hemp plant that has a naturally high level of Cannabidiol (CBD) compound present in its structure. Different Sativa plants are bred to yield those plants that have abundant Cannabidiol (CBD) and very low levels of tetrahydrocannabinol (THC). Tetrahydrocannabinol (THC) is one of the most commonly occurring cannabinoids in the Sativa plant, it is followed by Cannabidiol (CBD). There are more than 100 cannabinoids that have identified the Sativa plant. However, THC and CBD have been under the scrutiny of the scientific populace for many years for different reasons.

The natural precursor known as cannabigerolic acid (CBGA) in the Sativa plant is controlled by the naturally occurring enzyme called synthases. These synthases are the reason the sativa plant could differ and produce greater or lesser THC, CBD, or CBC. Industrial hemp has been tested to have higher levels of the recessive gene that could produce plants that have lower chances of THC production. That is why different breeds of sativa plant that are genetically inclined to have these recessive genes are cross-bred together to produce a plant that has more chances of having CBD-synthase enzyme and lesser THC-synthase.

Cannabidiol (CBD) does not cause the person ingesting it to become high, where its counterpart Tetrahydrocannabinol (THC) has been labeled to cause psychotropic effects after ingestion. Plants that have been bred to have a higher dose of the CBD-synthase are used to extract pure cannabidiol or concentrated CBD hemp oil. This particular cannabinoid oil has other nutritious elements as well such as terpenes, vitamins, amino acids, omega-3 fatty acids. Moreover, it may also contain other naturally occurring phytocannabinoids like cannabidivarin (CBCV), cannabinol (CBN), cannabigerol (CBG), and cannabichromene (CBD).

Over the years, the production of CBD hemp oil has changed to produce different doses in different forms. It can be found as drops, chewing gum, or in capsules. It may be applied as a topical ointment in pure concentrated forms. The concentrated pure hemp oil has higher chances of infusing into the skin to give many natural benefits.

CBD HEMP OIL DOSAGE: HOW TO TAKE IT AS A SUPPLEMENT?

CBD Hemp oil or CBD oil has been derived from those hemp plants that have higher levels of CBD. The seeds and stalks of this plant are jam-packed with hemp seed oil that has a high concentration of cannabidiol. Being a therapeutic medicine, it is given in various forms that could be added to the daily regiment to help with multiple issues. The intake of the CBD oil has been categorized into different types of products such:

- The CBD oil can be taken through oral applicators that have already been measured to help the individuals take the perfect amount. It is taken through the mouth and put under the tongue for the recommended amount of time, after which it is swallowed.
- The CBD Oil could be ingested by adding its liquid form into other foods or by adding it to a smoothie. The liquid is made to be concentrated so it may act as a supplement that can be taken as it is or by mixing it with other foods.

- Another popular form of CBD Oil supplements is oil capsules that are already measured to offer the perfect mix of vitamins during the daily regimen. It could easily be added to the daily morning supplement and vitamin routine.

- CBD Oil can also be found as a vaporizer; it can enter the blood-stream to offer instant relief to skin issues, digestive, and liver issues. It is one of the most efficient methods of taking CBD.

- The CBD hemp oil could also be found in specific food items that are specially designed to make the ingestion easier. They could be found as candies with added sweeteners to make the process far more fun and more comfortable.

- One of the most popular methods of application for CBD hemp oil is through topical treatment. This could be offered as soothing salves, balms, shampoos, conditioners, moisturizers, anti-aging skin care, body washes, and other things of similar nature.

CBD HEMP OIL BENEFITS: HOW GOOD IS IT FOR MY BODY?

The research done on the Sativa plant has led to many discoveries bringing many treatment remedies for various issues. The CBD Hemp Oil, in particular, has been hand-picked from natural growing sativa plants that have a high concentration of CBD Cannabinoid. This component of the sativa plant does not have the hallucinatory or psychoactive effects that are associated with cannabis. Instead, it gives all the beneficial effects that offer relief and nutrition to the individuals ingesting it. It has one of the most helpful qualities that help individuals medically and therapeutically. CBD Hemp oil could be used as:

- A digestive aid, it helps the body maintain a healthy stomach environment that would allow them to heal and prevent any illnesses. It increases the appetite for people that have issues digesting food and causing irreparable damage. The National Cancer Institute has researched the effects of CBD oil on the digestive system, they have found that CBD binds with the naturally occurring cannabinoids in the body to help it regulate and maintain a healthy feeding behavior. When Cannabidiol (CBD) is connected to the naturally occurring cannabinoid receptors, the body automatically behaves in a regular pattern of eating behavior. As a digestive aid, it could also help with vomiting and nausea that is caused by other illnesses or due to a digestive problem. One of the most common treatments for individuals that have endured chemotherapy and similar therapy would be CBD hemp oil, as it could help reduce nausea followed by the treatment.

- As an analgesic, there has been a lot of study of Cannabidiol (CBD) through which individuals have been given pain relief for nerve injury, chemotherapy, diabetes, and neuropathy. The CBD receptors have also found to help with inflammatory pain and swelling, which commonly occurs in chronic diseases. Specific diseases and the effect CBD Hemp Oil as an analgesic have been discussed in the next chapters.

- As a therapeutic medicine, regular use of CBD Hemp oil may also help individuals with anxiety disorders. Social anxiety disorder or generalized anxiety disorder is one of the most commonly occurring mental health disorder, which causes much discomfort in the daily lives of people. The most common method of treating this disorder is through medication and counseling that could take months to settle and give effects. However, CBD hemp oil could offer quicker relief with less adverse effects. CBD Hemp Oil has concentrated form of Cannabidiol (CBD), unlike marijuana that has higher levels of Tetrahydrocannabinol (THC). Due to the high concentration of THC, marijuana causes more chances of anxiety in individuals that already have anxiety disorders. A study conducted in 2011 showed that people who took regular CBD hemp oil had a significant decrease in cognitive impairment, discomfort during a speech, and anxiety. This research gave half the participants placebo pills, while half were given CBD oil. Those who were given the placebo pills still exhibited anxiety and stress during social situations.

- As an antipsychotic medicine, CBD oil can also relieve the psychotic symptoms felt during schizophrenic episodes. The University of Cologne in Germany has done extensive research on the effects of regular use of this oil on people with psychotic disorders, which has been discussed in later chapters.

- For the management of cancer pain, many cannabinoids exiting the body and those that exist in nature have been under the scope of research for many years. The cannabinoid receptors found in Cannabidiol (CBD) have been shown to offer relief through peripheral and systematic routes. However, this research is still an ongoing preclinical study, where CB-1 and CB-2 (CBD receptors) could be used for pain modulation.

CBD HEMP OIL AND ITS SIDE EFFECTS THROUGH MISUSE

Some studies have shown that diluted hemp oil that has not been adequately processed or picked for its concentrated CBD cannabinoid could show an adverse effect. Traces of THC cannabinoid may cause the individual taking it a momentary high. It may also irritate individuals with mental health disorders. As THC is known to have lasting effects on the brain and behavior of adults and adolescents. It could contribute to psychotic issues in mental health patients, which may affect through further heightening of psychotic features existing with the disorder. The hemp oil that has not been adequately checked for THC content may also cause individuals that regularly take it as a supplement to develop the amotivational syndrome.

This syndrome could cause lowered cognition abilities, lack of activity, incoherence, and apathy. Higher dosage of THC cannabinoid does not impose any danger when ingested for a short-time period. However, long-term use may cause psychopathological problems. If used for recreational purposes, this type of unrefined hemp oil may also cause the individuals taking it regularly to develop withdrawal syndrome that is associated with anxiety, yawning, tiredness, and depression. The THC cannabinoid has also been reported to cause impairment of motor skills due to the incoordination of the cerebellar. This incoordination is similar to that which is caused by alcohol products.

Nonetheless, if the CDB hemp oil is taken from trusted marketers, there should be no problem ingesting this oil on a regular basis. It will not cause any psychotic or hallucinatory effects during regular use. Instead, it would have the nutritional effects of hemp oil and the therapeutic effects of the CBD that could help with many issues and diseases that affect physically or mentally. In the next chapter, the usage and effects of CBD oil on individuals with specific illness has been explained in detail. This help individuals interested in adding CBD hemp oil as a regular supplement find the right amount and the right way to ingest CBD in their daily lives.

CHAPTER TWO - PHYSICAL BENEFITS OF CBD HEMP OIL

The physical and nutritional benefits of CBD Hemp oil range from high to lows, it acts as a remedy for many common issues such as insomnia and stomach issues to acute problems such as diabetes. CBD Hemp oil does not have any psychoactive effects that are exhibited in marijuana, which has been shunned by the society even though it has a better side for a healthy living. On the other hand, CBD hemp oil has all the best sides of marijuana and almost no adverse effects if taken as advised. Individuals cannot overdose with CBD oil products, whose common factor is CBD cannabinoid. Moreover, it also counters some of the adverse effects of THC cannabinoid-like lethargy, memory loss, paranoia, intoxication, and tachycardia.

Before going into depth about different illnesses; the CBD Hemp oil benefits and dosage by the diseases, we must understand the (ECS) endocannabinoid system associated with it. The endocannabinoid system is a newly discovered system that is present in all mammals. It is made up of hundreds and thousands of cannabinoid receptors, whose site location is in the brain, central nervous system, and the immune system. The CB1 receptor moves through the central nervous system, and the CB2 receptors move through the immune system.

The human body does have the ability to produce its cannabinoid; surprisingly, it does not have to depend upon plants for these receptor cannabinoids. It has cannabinoids such as 2-AG, Anandamide, and CBD, which help the body cells communicate with each other to make sure that all the body functions are behaving normally. However, most of the times people do not care for this system that plays a significant role in supporting and maintain the health of our body.

CBD HEMP OIL AS A BONE STIMULANT

CBD Hemp oil has many components that can help with bone issues; it can also help develop better communication of the (ECS) endocannabinoid system in the affected areas. Research has also shown that cannabinoids present in CBD oil can help bone metabolism through regulation. It was also concluded that if the CB1 receptors in the human body were at low concentration, then they could have impaired bone activity and formation. On the other hand, if there is a deficiency of CB2 receptors in the body, then there is a chance for the individuals to develop age-related bone disorders like osteoporosis. (8)

Above all, some cannabinoids also help with the development and maintenance of synovial tissue, or in simpler words the maintenance of the tissue surrounding the bones. The damage to synovial tissue due to lower cannabinoid concentration could cause inflammatory arthritis. Let us see the effects of CBD Hemp oil on bone-related issues and diseases in detail.

OSTEOPOROSIS

Osteoporosis is one of the most common diseases that occur in the skeleton system of the human body. This disease occurs when there is a miscommunication of the receptors in the area due to unhealthy conditions of the (ECS) endocannabinoid system. However, it may also happen with age. Osteoporosis may cause the body to create too little bone or too much bone in the area; this causes the bones to become weak. Weak bones could easily be damaged or injured by a minor fall or through bumping into objects.

By the miscommunication in the ECS system, it may also be caused due to other deficiencies or issues such immune disorders and digestive problems. CBD Hemp oil could treat this miscommunication as it has beneficial cannabinoids that could help with the maintenance of bone. CBD Hemp oil contains cannabinoids such as CBD, CBC, CBG, and THC(V) that could help individuals with osteoporosis with regular use.

OSTEOARTHRITIS

Being a degenerative disease, it causes pain and inflammation that affects the bones and joint cartilages of the body. This disease could cause pain in the knee, hip and thumb joints. This issue could be treated by offering the (ECS) endocannabinoid system of the body cannabinoids such as CBD, CBG, CBC, CBG (A), and CBD (A). These cannabinoids are found in CBD Hemp oil in abundance; it helps people with osteoarthritis relief from the constant pain as it is an anti-inflammatory oil.

RHEUMATOID ARTHRITIS (RA):

Inflammation categorizes this disease in the joints as the body attacks these the joints and bone tissue due to a mistake by the immune system of the body. Long-term damage to this disease may cause the bone to deform and erode over time. This disease could be treated by introducing cannabinoids such as CBD, CBG, CBC, CBG (A), CGC (A), THC (A), and CBD (A). These cannabinoids are present CBD rich hemp oil that is why it is suggested that it could treat and bring relief to individuals with Rheumatoid arthritis through regular use.

USE OF CDB HEMP OIL FOR BONE DISORDER AND DISEASES

Many clinical studies in 2014, 2015, and 2017 by professionals of pharmacology and anesthesia have been made that suggest that CBD oil could treat inflammation issues and relieve pain in joint related diseases. (9) In these research experiments, the participants that were given CBD Hemp oil topical treatment and CBD oil pill regularly to reach this conclusion. By those research conclusions, diseases like osteoporosis, osteoarthritis, and Rheumatoid arthritis (RA) could be treated through a topical application on the affected areas after regular intervals.

CDB hemp oil is found in gel and cream form that could be applied in the affected areas regularly during the daily massage sessions. It could also be taken in capsule form that contains a high concentration of CBD in the hemp oil so it would have maximum effect on the body.

CBD HEMP OIL AS ANTI-BACTERIAL AND ANTI-PSORIATIC

Skin health is one of the most common queries of people that struggle with acne and other skin conditions. This deviation in the skin is due to weak blood flow and regenerative skin conditions that could cause further skin conditions. CBD Hemp Oil can be used to treat many skin conditions due to the presence of skin-friendly cannabinoids that help the skin become healthier and smoother.

Some facialists in Manhattan have also claimed that CBD oil is "the argan oil of the future." This is due to the anti-inflammatory, anti-acne, anti-bacterial, and anti-psoriatic abilities of this oil. No wonder, it is claimed as the next best thing for various skin conditions. The CBD present in the oil could also help regenerate skin cells quicker regarding a skin wound. The anti-inflammatory cannabinoids present in the oil have very powerful abilities that soothe irritated skins cells. Philip Blair, who is a renown medical advisor, has also claimed that it could outperform the healing abilities of vitamin D and C for skin conditions. It could give the much-needed cannabinoid balance to the endocannabinoid system (ECS) for healthier skin.

ACNE

Most acne forms such as adult acne are due to inflammation of the skin because the skin barrier has been compromised. When this barrier is weakened bacteria, and fatty-acid could cause the area to become inflamed, this could further cause hyperpigmentation. The skin health depends upon the endocannabinoid system (ECS) of the body, which regulates and maintains important systems. If there is an imbalance of this system, it could cause various issues that are taken care by the ECS.

CBD Hemp oil has powerful anti-bacterial and anti-inflammatory abilities that provide balance to the skin and maintains a healthy skin barrier that prevents further acne. Hemp oil also contains terpenes that have anti-septic and sebum-reducing abilities, which further contributes to keeping the skin healthy. CBD Hemp has cannabinoids like CBD, CBG, CBC (A), SBG (A), and CBD (A) that contribute to the anti-inflammatory, antibacterial, and antiseptic properties.

ECZEMA

Eczema is a skin disorder that causes the skin to become red and itchy; it may flare up due to weather or allergy. It may cause the skin to become patchy or cracked in areas. This skin disorder has no cure so far. However, many potential skin medicines could help reduce the condition significantly. The irregular behavior of the endocannabinoid system due to an imbalance of natural receptors could cause the skin to misbehave. This imbalance of receptors may cause conditions such as eczema to develop over time.

Through clinical trial and research, it was found out that the cannabinoid receptor agonists in CBD Hemp oil could reduce the itching sensation caused by eczema. This reduction in itching is made by activation of anhidrotic nerve fibers and production of neuropeptide by the cannabinoid receptors present in the CBD Hemp Oil. The pro-inflammatory mediators were significantly reduced by the introduction of cannabinoids such CBD, CBG, CBC (A), SBG (A), and CBD (A) that are readily present in CBD Hemp Oil.

PSORIASIS

Psoriasis causes multiple skin issues due to the overproduction of skin cells. It causes the skin underneath the excess cells to become inflamed and sometimes, infected with bacteria. This disease is caused by internal deficiencies and is further irritated by external mismanagement. Most of the treatment for this disease only deal with the inside deficiencies or the outside skin conditions. Rarely, some expensive treatments are available that could expertly handle both conditions as one.

However, CBD hemp oil is an affordable method to treat psoriasis due to its anti-psoriatic abilities as well as many other skin-friendly effects. These effects range from dealing with inflamed and irritated skin areas and the removal of bacteria from the weakened skin. The CBD has a skin-calming effect when it is regularly used. The CBD cannabinoid itself acts as an antipsoriatic, anti-inflammatory, and anti-bacterial component to deal with many skin conditions.

SKIN WOUNDS

Those skin wounds that are caused by painful skin conditions such as melanoma can also be treated with CBD Hemp oil could provide relief to the wounded areas as it has pain relieving properties. Many other conditions that are interconnected with skin wounds such as skin infection and inflammation can also be dealing with the regular usage of CBD hemp oil. This oil has also be reported to give instant relief through topical treatment according to a report article posted by The Journal of Pain and Management.

SCALP CARE

Scalp, being one of the most sensitive areas, can become easily irritated to cause issues such as dandruff and dryness. This dryness could further provoke the hair follicles to behave in an irregular manner and lo and behold; hair fall becomes one of the lists of problems to deal with as well. This dryness could be combatted by giving the scalp proper hydration through the use of CBD hemp oil conditioner and shampoos.

CBD Hemp oil has omega-3 and omega-6 fatty acids that create an optimal environment for the scalp to enhance and protect the skin of your scalps. The human body cannot make omega-6 fatty acid that anti-inflammatory properties, however, not all omega-6 fatty acids have this property. The fatty acids found in CBD Oil can soothe the irritated areas of the skin and help to treat conditions such as hyper epidermal proliferation. Through regular use of CBD hemp oil hair products, the scalp can develop a healthier skin barrier, which allows it to become flexible and moisturized.

USE OF CDB HEMP OIL FOR SKIN CONDITIONS AND WOUNDS

CBD hemp oil has many cannabinoids that boost the endocannabinoid system (ECS) of the body; it allows them to perform better to give a healthier skin system. The CBD hemp oil has many properties such as antiseptic, anti-bacterial, anti-inflammatory, and so forth, which could help through topical applications. Oral ingestion of pills could help inherent deficiencies of the system.

Furthermore, the hemp oil also contains healthy fatty acids such as omega-6 and omega-3 that supports the hair and skin growths. It offers many benefits along with nutritional contents that keep the skin healthy and happy through regular usage. CBD Hemp oil is available as balms and creams that could be applied to the affected skin to treat many conditions such as acne, eczema, and so forth. The scalp conditions can also be maintained by moisturizing and shampooing with CBD enriched shampoos that are known to combat dryness.

More importantly, CBD Hemp oil balms are enriched with nutrients of the hemp oil and the CBD concentrate that contains minerals, proteins, and fatty acids. The nutrient content of hemp oil and the beneficial properties of CBD can help the skin maintain a healthy skin barrier. The CBD hemp oil can also be taken through tinctures and topical creams that should be considered as advised on the packaging as different companies have different concentration of CBD in the products.

CBD HEMP OIL AS AN IMMUNOSUPPRESSIVE

The immune system of the body can be balanced through the regular use of CBD Hemp Oil. Research has shown that many cannabinoids that are present in CBD hemp oil can balance the immune system so that it performs in a regular and healthier manner. The cannabinoids found in the CBD hemp oil can act as a neuromodulator to modulate the immune response. The endocannabinoid system (ECS) plays a significant part in regulating the behavior of the immune system. It creates a link between healthy the immune system and the cannabinoids so that the body can recover from self-imposed inflammatory diseases.

The cannabinoids present in CBD hemp oil can promote behavior of neural pathways and allow the construction of new ones. Moreover, it also reduces the inflammation caused by the immune system that can help balance its functions. Primarily, the two functions that can be effected through the ECS are the Cell-Mediated Immunity and Humoral Immunity. The former is responsible for the creation of phagocytes (antigen-specific T-lymphocytes) that helps restore and neutralize any threats into body make it behave normally, while, the later uses macromolecules to fight against antigens (foreign toxins or substances that causes the immune system to act).

All in all, CBD hemp oil has many properties that could balance the immune system of the body with the help of the endocannabinoid system (ECS). It also can offer pain relief as many of the diseases caused by the immune system have symptoms of progressive pain.

MULTIPLE SCLEROSIS

Being a chronic neurological disease, multiple sclerosis has been under the microscope of scientist for many years. It is a complex disease that is caused by the autoimmune system of the body, the most common symptoms of this disease encompass muscle spasm, stiffness, fatigue, bladder and bowel issues, severe pain, fatigue, cognitive changes, spasticity, and many other of the like. The research to find a treatment for this chronic disease is ongoing; it has no permanent cure. However, many safe and effective management medicines could reverse the damage and combat further abuse of the body.

The Cannabinoids present in CBD hemp oil are known to improve pain, spasticity, and inflammations. It has immunomodulatory and inflammatory properties that help in the treatment of MS through regular usage. It has a combination of cannabinoids that help modulate the neural pathways through pharmacological activity, which can decrease the inflammatory effects of the cells. MS also causes the immune-mediated inflammatory response, which it cannot be dealt with ordinary methods of treatment. Research has shown that it could be due to "counter-regulatory mechanisms used to heal injured tissue" (9)

Nonetheless, CBD can mitigate this condition by providing targeted treatment through the cannabinoids present in its constituents. To put it simply, allows the inflammation of the pathways to go down through downregulation of proteins, while also reducing the spastic conditions caused by it. CBD hemp oil is also known for its analgesic properties that could significantly reduce the pain felt by this progressive disease.

LUPUS

Lupus is another very dangerous autoimmune disease that causes the immune system to behave irregularly. The immune system of the body attacks its tissue by mistake; it considers this tissue as virus or bacteria. This disease could be caused by the changes in the environment, genetics, or hormones. The most common symptoms that categorize this disease are skin rashes, inflammation, mood swings, soreness, hair loss, anemia, heart problems, fatigue and so forth. This disease itself is not harmful, however, if not treated or appropriately mediated can cause further problems in the kidney or heart.

One of the most common categorizations of lupus is inflammation that is caused by the attack on healthy tissues. This effect can be reduced through CBD hemp oil as it has very powerful anti-inflammatory effects through regular dosage. Concentrated CBD has CB-2 receptors that help the endocannabinoid system (ECS) regulate and maintain normal inflammatory responses. Various strains of CBD hemp oil can also help alleviate the inflammatory responses by increasing the concentration of anti-inflammatory proteins in the body. CBD hemp oil has many cannabinoids that have anti-inflammatory, analgesic, anorectic properties that can deal with the common issues caused by lupus.

CANCER

Autoimmunity in the body causes the immune system to attack or remove tissues in the body when it has found something foreign or toxic in the body. This is known as the Th1 response of the immune system. However, it can misbehave when it cannot differentiate between the organism and the toxin. Let us suppose; the kidney has stored some toxic matters ingested in fat cells of the body. In this case, when the immune system has a Th1 response to these toxins that have merged with the body could cause it to turn against the healthy fat cells as well. If there is an imbalance in the immune system that has produced repression of the Th1 system, then the death of the useless cells in the body will be hindered. This slowed down the response of the immune system would lead to a build-up of unnecessarily and useless cells that could cause cancer over a period.

CBD Hemp oil has the necessary cannabinoid receptors that could balance the irregularities in the immune system to moderate the inflammation caused by it. The CBD, CBG, CBC, THC (A), and CBD (A) cannabinoids present in CBD-rich hemp oil has anti-proliferative abilities that can inhibit the growth of cancer/tumor cells. The studies done by National Cancer Institute have also claimed that CBD concentrate or CBD hemp oil can have anti-tumor effects. The clinical research conducted by National Cancer Institute suggests that it "may have a protective effect against the development of certain types of tumors." Another study has stated that the regular intake of CBD hemp oil can decrease the involvement of the gene responsible for breast cancer. The CBD cannabinoid controls the tumor cells by inhibiting their growth and inducing death.

USE OF CDB HEMP OIL FOR AUTOIMMUNE DISEASES

CBD Hemp Oil is found in various forms and can have different strains that have processed to give specific effects. For illnesses as acute as autoimmune disorders, it is essential that you talk to doctor before taking it as a supplement. To get best results for diseases such as lupus, multiple sclerosis, and cancer, it would be best if the CBD hemp oil is of high quality.

The CBD hemp oil made from industrial hemp may not have enough concentration of CBD to effect the disorders as a quality one would. It may also have other chemical derivatives that cause further damage to the body. If the CBD hemp oil is taken as a tincture, then it can be diluted with other nutritional oils such as olive oil or coconut oil.

The best way to take tinctures is to hold them under the tongue for about two to three minutes before swallowing. High-quality CBD hemp has therapeutic cannabinoids that could enter through the tongue into the bloodstream. After consulting with the doctor, CBD hemp oil could also be used as a mouth spray, which has an average dose of eight to twelve times. Many strains of CBD hemp oil can also be used as a targeted treatment for Multiple Sclerosis, which will be discussed in later chapters.

Other modes of consumption and application for CBD hemp oil are the transdermal patch, vaporized CBD oil, CBD rich edibles, CBD hemp oil capsules, tinctures, drinks, and topical. Each of these forms varies in CB concentration due to manufacturing differences and sativa plant breeding techniques that is why it is important to find the best-suited form by taking small dosages. More importantly, it is best to take vaporized CBD oil to relieve pain symptoms associated with the disease. The CBD enriched edibles should be consumed at night, so it may work along with the body's self-repair system to keep the pain and inflammation at bay.

CBD HEMP OIL AS AN ANTI-DIABETIC

Numerous research sessions have been conducted to find the various health benefits of CBD Hemp oil. So far, it has been concluded that the cannabinoids present in the CBD-enriched hemp oil can be beneficial for some disorders and diseases, including diabetes. Being one of the most common diseases in the world, diabetes has affected millions of people. Diabetes is caused by insulin and insulin resistance of the body; it causes the blood to have high levels of sugar/ glucose. Diabetes is generated when the body does not produce insulin properly that is associated with the decrease in blood glucose.

The CBD cannabinoid present in the CBD hemp oil plays a vital role in the chronic inflammation that is categorized in type 2 diabetes, it could offer relief and reduction in the inflammation. Being an anti-inflammatory and anti-diabetic, CBD hemp oil has become one of the primary focus of scientists dealing with the treatment of diabetes. Chief Executive Officer Mark J. Rosenfeld working at ISA Scientific has also stated that "Unlike insulin and other existing medications for diabetes, CBD may actually suppress, reverse and perhaps cure the disease," which leads us to believe that it could control and develop healthier body systems through regular usage, unlike momentary relief from the traditional methods of medication.

Additionally, research on mice has also shown that regular CBD hemp oil dosage can also decrease the risk of developing diabetes from 83% to 30%. (10) Furthermore, other clinical studies have also shown that individuals that use CBD Hemp oil as a supplement in their daily regiment have lower fasting insulin levels, which present at higher levels could cause diabetic conditions. Let us see in detail how CBD hemp oil works on the different types of diabetes.

TYPE 1 DIABETES

This type of diabetes stems from the categorization of irregular insulin behavior, which is caused by an autoimmune attack. This type of diabetes is commonly seen in individuals under the age of thirty. However, it can be diagnosed in older adults as well.

Approximately, 86 million people are prediabetes; this could be handled if appropriately treated. Yet, most individuals do not know about their pre-diabetic symptoms. It causes the immune system to attack the pancreas's islet cells. This causes the pancreases to produce very low levels of insulin and sometimes no insulin. The symptoms associated with type 1 diabetes are thirst, extreme hunger, weight loss, mood changes, weakness, frequent urination, blurred vision, among other things.

The cannabinoids present in CBD hemp oil can help maintain a healthy Endocannabinoid System (ECS), which can play an important role in keeping diabetic and pre-diabetic in-check. The CB1 receptors present in the CBD hemp oil can help increase the insulin secretion in some cases. Moreover, it also demonstrates analgesic qualities to relieve pain and as a by-product reduce oxidative stress. Being anti-inflammatory in effects, it can help reduce symptoms such as inflammation associated with diabetes. It also has a positive impact on the metabolism of the body that restores homeostasis balance leading to the regular mode of operation. By bringing balance to the homeostasis system, the body can act on its own to produce natural healing abilities. Ongoing research has reported that CBD hemp oil cannot prevent type 1 diabetes. However, it can reduce the complications associated with this illness.

CBD hemp oil can help regulate the vascular inflammation, atherosclerosis (build-up of plaque in arteries), and oxidative stress to manage cardiovascular complications. It can thicken and expand the glomerular membrane that helps with diabetic nephropathy. It also reduces the risk of blindness in adults as the lower levels of cannabinoid receptors are located in the retina. CBD hemp oil can alleviate the lower levels of CB1 receptors that would prevent the death of retinal cells. These receptors also help with the damage caused by long-term hyperglycemia, which causes painful sensory neuron stimulation in case of diabetic neuropathy.

TYPE 2 DIABETES

Type 2 diabetes is commonly diagnosed in individuals over the age of forty or those individuals that are obese. It is categorized by the insulin resistance as well as irregular insulin production. This causes the blood glucose levels in the body to rise higher causing multiple complications. Type 2 Diabetes is also known as hyperglycemia, which is one of the most commonly occurring diabetic diseases.

Type 2 diabetes is associated with insulin resistance; it is caused when the body rejects the naturally produce insulin, which is responsible for regulating the glucose metabolism. The body becomes resistant to insulin. In this case; it refuses the glucose carried by it. In turn, the glucose starts to build up in the body to develop a condition known as hyperglycemia. Furthermore, the individuals that have type 2 diabetes also experience nerve damage in the areas such as feet and hand to cause numbness and pain.

CBD hemp oil is shown to reduce the amount of blood glucose in the body, as well as the inflammation caused by the insulin resistance. The anti-inflammatory properties found in CBD hemp oil can also improve metabolism through regular use.

A research done by the University of California has shown that individuals using CBD hem oil regularly as a supplement had reduced symptoms in their pre-diabetic symptoms in those that had it and lowered the blood sugar levels in all. In the like manner, another clinical research report by the American Journal of Medicine also concluded that there were residual effects of CBD oil usage on people that had used it at least once. It had caused lower levels of the fasting insulin as well as the insulin resistance factor (IR). Coupled with this conclusion, it can be deemed that through the regular use of CDB hemp oil, there is a chance that the type-2 diabetic symptoms can be controlled and regulated, if not completely removed.

OBESITY

Weight gain is very closely related to diabetes, as it is an effect and cause of this disease. Various clinical research sessions have been conducted to find out the effects of CBD hemp oil on diabetic patients that struggle with obesity. Concentrated CBD hemp oil can help individuals with diabetes have a faster loss of weight, whereas, there is a chance that the weight of the pancreas may increase. The cannabinoids found in CBD hemp oil can protect the beta cells found in the pancreas, which may also lead to regulated behavior of the immune system in type 1 diabetes.

DIABETIC RETINOPATHY

After a period, struggling with diabetes, patients often develop a co-occurring disease known as diabetic retinopathy. This disease acts as a complication associated with diabetes as the cells in the retina, particularly the Cannabinoid receptors, become damaged over a period. This damage becomes irreparable as the blood-retinal barrier has permanent breakdowns that prevent blood flow in the retinal tissue. The breakdown categorized by this complication is due to the glucose that causes exposure of neurotoxins in the neural tissue. There is also a chance that the damage to the neural tissue may cause bleeding.

CBD hemp oil can be used to avoid such a complication as it has been studied to show positive results. The CBD causes a reduction in the oxidative stress and nontoxicity of the neural tissue; this allows the blood-retinal barrier to become stronger and have a less chance of breakdown. The CBD cannabinoid also prevents the retinal cells from dying.

USE OF CDB HEMP OIL FOR DIABETIC DISEASES

Diabetic patients can add CBD hemp oil as a regular supplement to their diet as it would have more beneficial effects than adverse ones. Having many other cannabinoid constituents along with a high concentration of CBD cannabinoid in the CBD hemp oil can offer many benefits to a diabetic patient. CBD hemp oil has anti-inflammatory, anti-diabetic, analgesic, and immunosuppressive that allows it to deal with the symptoms of diabetes and prevent further degradation of the system.

The oil used for acute conditions such as diabetes should have a high concentration of CBD, it also should be taken from naturally grown hemp plants to avoid further contamination of chemicals. One of the most concentrated forms is found in tinctures that should be held under the tongue for two to three minutes; it allows the nutrients to be carried into the bloodstream efficiently.

As an addition to the supplement routine, CBD hemp oil can be taken in the form of capsules/pills or as additives to food items such as candies or gummies. The CBD hemp oil may remain in your digestive system and give relief for six to seven hours if taken orally.

For the immediate relief of pain, CBD hemp oil should be applied topically to the areas of concern. It could be used as a vaporizer for a smoother transition of the cannabinoids into the bloodstream. This type of method can last up to three to four hours depending upon the CBD Concentrate. The swelling in the joints like finger joints and wrist could also be reduced by apply topical CBD hemp oil on the skin such as balms and creams.

CBD HEMP OIL AS AN ANALGESIC

CBD Hemp Oil provides a helping hand to the endocannabinoid system to offer non-euphoriant pain relief and management. It acts on a molecular level with the help of the cannabinoid receptors to provide modulation and regulation of various systems of the body. As a pleiotropic drug, it can affect many systems of the body through the molecular pathways. The concentration of the CBD cannabinoid plays an essential role in activating the serotonin receptors to offer therapeutic effects as well.

CBD cannabinoid in the oil is also responsible for preventing the absorption of anandamide into the body that is responsible for managing pain. The abundance of anandamide in the body significantly reduces the amount of pain felt by a person as it constantly moves into the bloodstream. Moreover, it also reduces the inflammation caused by the nervous system and the brain through its anti-inflammatory abilities.

The effects of CBD hemp oil for the management of pain provided instant relief in the muscles and joints through proper application. The active and natural ingredients present in the hemp oil gives it many attributes that help the body deal with various issues at once.

CHRONIC PAIN

The manifestation of pain in various parts of the body has become one of the most common symptoms associated with various diseases. This type of pain does not give a cautious time limit to the patients; rather, they have to endure the pain for many years until they find a viable treatment. Most of the traditional pain management's medicine for chronic pain has many side effects, which may cause other complications to brew in the body.

CBD hemp oil, being a non-psychotropic compound, can help individuals find relief from the pain without the adverse effects of marijuana. The CBD hemp oil taken from naturally grown plants have a full spectrum of compounds that pull at each other to provide even more beneficial results. This effects of magnifying each other's powers are known as the entourage effect, where the whole body benefits through a process called homeostasis. The regular use of CBD hemp oil causes the body to become active and find less suffering. Clinical studies have shown that the rostral anterior cingulate cortex (AC) manages the emotions felt over pain. When CBD hemp oil is introduced into the rAAC system, then the sensations of pain could be diminished.

CBD hemp oil can also be used to diminish pain felt through chronic inflammation. Bringing to notice, the anti-inflammatory properties of the oil, it can be safely said the reduction of the inflammation was imminent result through regular use. Another research done on the rats also concluded that the neuropathic pain that was triggered due to chronic nerve constrictions could be managed by administrating regular dosage of CBD hemp oil. The results of the management of chronic pain were evident after two weeks of regular use, where pain sensations were reduced in various thermal conditions.

Identically, it can be said that the cannabinoids such as CBD, CBN, CBC, and CBG (A) would reduce the chronic and inflammatory pain felt by a human through regular use. CBD hemp oil is a more comfortable alternative to manage these kind pains as well as those felt during injuring. This oil has also been used to manage the chronic pain's felt by the cancer patient, which reported that it was a manageable alternative with little to no side effects.

BACK PAIN

Back Pain is another chronic pain condition that is caused by inflammation of the muscles or back. This condition causes the patient to ingest a significant amount of medication. The reason for the amount of pain caused by this condition is due to its relation to the nerve fibers in the back. It could also cause the patient to become uncomfortable enough to develop anxiety or depressive disorders. The anti-inflammatory properties of the muscle relaxant taken for this pain create many other adverse conditions such as gastrointestinal disorder, cramps, constipation, and stomach ulcers.

When the intervertebral discs in the spinal cord become weak, then there a massive amount of neck and back pain. It could be caused by irregular water and sugar levels, oxygen deficiency, inflammation, and aging, and various other issues of the like. Research has also shown that the Intervertebral Disc Degeneration in patients could be handled by the protective effects of CBD hemp oil, particularly the CBD cannabinoid.

This study further instigated that the lower dosages of CBD hemp oil had no effects on the individuals that took it. However, high concentrated CBD hemp oil revealed a significant increase in the healing of the damaged intervertebral disc. The CBD hemp oil was labeled to have anti-degenerative effects when taken in concentration.

FIBROMYALGIA

Fibromyalgia is categorized by the pain that is felt in various parts of the body such as the skeletal tissue and muscles. Recently, this condition was labeled as a chronic disease, whereas, in the past, it was diagnosed as a syndrome, commonly known as the Yuppie Flu. This disease causes the fibers in the body to report sensations of pain to the brain from all over the body. One of the possible causes of this issue has been identified as stress, where the extreme situations may cause a flare-up. It has also been studies that females might be more susceptible to have this condition.

Usually, patients that suffer from this condition have very low tolerance for pain; they may also suffer from other disorders such as Chronic Fatigue Syndrome,

IBS, and Migraine. The pain regulatory system of the body can be managed by alleviating the certain cannabinoids found in the body; these cannabinoids can help the body with the assistance of the Endocannabinoid system. The receptors used by this system can provide potential relief to the individuals who have fibromyalgia. CBD cannabinoid reduces the cytokine count of the body that leads to reduced inflammation and pain.

Two of the most discussed beneficial effects of CBD hemp oil is that it is an analgesic and anti-inflammatory medicine. These properties allow the Endocannabinoid system to perform better and become regulated. This system controls many other parts of the body, and a deficiency in this system could cause pain and other issues. Fibromyalgia that is caused by such a deficiency can be managed by providing the Endocannabinoid system necessary constituents by using CBD hemp oil as a treatment.

MIGRAINES

Migraines usually cause excruciating pain when there is an attack; it causes many other issues that are as uncomfortable as the main issue itself. The conditions caused by migraine range from an earache, dizzy spells, nausea, double vision, vertigo, and other related problems. The biggest concern related to migraines is that it does not have any permanent cure. However, there are many medical prescriptions available to treat symptoms associated with it.

Recently, a journal published in the 'Pharmacotherapy' stated that the frequency of migraines could be significantly lowered through the use of CBD oil. This conclusion was based on a study that included 120 patients out which 100 patients were seen to have decreased in the frequency of the migraine attacks. However, three of them suffered the migraine attack more often than usual. Several surveys have been conducted that show that the regular use of CBD hemp oil reduced the pain and inflammation caused by various issues including a migraine.

The cause of a migraine is related to the deficiency of the endocannabinoid system, which has the job of maintaining a healthy environment for the whole body. It is vital that this system receives the care needed for it to be in optimal conditions. This could be done by using CBD hemp oil as a supplement regularly. Moreover, the nutrient and the therapeutic effects of the body cause a relaxation effect on individuals that lowers the risk of migraine attacks. The National Institute on Drug Abuse has even claimed that they have not found any harmful effects of using CBD hemp oil as a supplement.

MENSTRUAL CRAMPS

Menstrual Cramps have become one of the most recurring pains that a woman feels in her life, they have to face this pain alone and wait it out until it has completed its regular cycle. The constant aches and discomfort associated with periods have become one the most irritable condition as of yet. Women have been struggling for ages to find a medicine that could alleviate the pain associated with periods. Even Queen

Victoria herself used CB products to lessen the pain that comes with menstrual cramps.

Taking ibuprofen regularly to relieve the pain can cause adverse effects on the liver and other parts of the body. However, CBD hemp oil can offer the same analgesic properties with the adverse effects. It even provides other nutritional benefits that can clear out the skin breakouts that happen to be a by-product of monthly periods. The analgesic properties in the CBD hemp oil are carried by the CB1 and CB2 receptors, granted that the endocannabinoid system in the uterus cells, then they provide pain relief as well as calming properties.

USE OF CDB HEMP OIL FOR CHRONIC PAIN AND RELATED ISSUES

The beauty of CBD hemp oil begins with its multi-treatment properties and its connection with the endocannabinoid system. This system uses endogenous cannabinoids present in the body to manage and maintain systems such as the nervous system, the immune system, etc. If this there is any deficiency of the cannabinoid receptors in the endocannabinoid system than there will adverse effects in the body.

As this system works on a molecular level and travels through various molecular pathways that are present in the skin, the blood, anywhere that it is supposed to manage. That is why it is more comfortable with the application or ingestion of CBD hemp oil. It can be absorbed into the bloodstream through vaporization for instant relief. However, these vapors lose their potency over the period of 1 to two hours. The CBD hemp oil pills have a higher chance of staying in the bloodstream provide more extended relief from pain.

Topical treatment is advised because it is easier to handle and apply for pain felt during a period or a migraine attack. The cannabinoid receptors get absorbed into the skin to provide an analgesic effect by connecting with the body's endocannabinoid system. The anti-inflammatory abilities of this will also soothe the irritated and inflamed areas that are causing the pain.

There are many strains and concentrations of CBD hemp oil that can be useful to treat chronic pains such as back pain and fibromyalgia. One of the best and most popular strains that can help with chronic issues is Charlotte's Web. However, there are other types of strains that have particular effects like uplifting the spirit, for headaches, for relaxation, or for more clarity. The difference between these CBD hemp oil strains is that they may have some other cannabinoid factors deluding the ratio of the oil. The difference of the strains may also depend upon the phenotype of the parent plant, which is the environment in which the plant brought. Different environments can pull out different cannabinoid constituents from the sciatica plant, even if the concentration of CBD is high. Other well-known CBD hemp oil strains are the sour tsunami and Harlequin; they may have some concentration THC cannabinoid. Further detail of the ration and effects of the THC content in these strains have been given in later chapters.

CBD HEMP OIL AS INTESTINAL ANTI-PROKINETIC AND APPETITE STIMULANT

CBD hemp oil has some benefits for stomach related issues such as eating disorders or gastritis. CBD hemp oil does not have any psychoactive effects on the body. However, it does have many other beneficial effects associated with its popular counterpart marijuana. CBD hemp oil has many medicinal and therapeutic effects on the body to help as a digestive aid. According to the National Cancer Institute, the illnesses that affect the digestive system can reduce a person's appetite to diminish completely.

The CBD cannabinoid stimulates the appetite by binding the cannabinoid receptors to the body. These receptors make the endocannabinoid system stronger, which can contribute to a stronger boost in overall health. These receptors play an important part in maintaining and regulating the health of the digestive system. These receptors can stimulate appetite when they are in abundance in the body.

Moreover, being a powerful analgesic can also contribute to its Anti-prokinetic properties. The CB1 Receptors, in particular, can relieve the pain caused by various stomach issues. This receptor also reduces inflammation in the areas that have been inflamed due to some disease.

GASTRITIS

This disease is caused when the stomach lining of the body is inflamed; it could develop into acute or chronic gastritis. Gastritis can develop in the body due to the infection of a bacteria known as Helicobacter pylori or through nonsteroidal anti-inflammatory medicine. Some of the other causes of gastritis are Crohn's disease, autoimmune issues, or sarcoidosis. The symptoms associated with this disease can range from bloating, indigestion, vomiting, nausea, abdominal pain, among others. Individuals with this disease may develop other severe conditions such as gastric cancer, peptic ulcer, anemia, MALT lymphoma, and structures that could lead to death.

This disease can be maintained by avoiding some food and chemicals that irritate the bowel and stomach area. Cigarette smoking could cause other stomach issues like indigestion that could further irritate the condition. An excessive amount of drinking and consuming alcohol can weaken the stomach that could cause other bacteria to infect it. Carbonated drinks, decaffeinated, and caffeinated drinks can also irritate the stomach lining of the body. Drinks that contain citric acid with deteriorating the condition, it may become acute in some cases.

Gastritis patients should eat foods that would hinder the growth of Helicobacter pylori bacteria; this could be food that has fiber and flavonoids. Some of the foods that should be consumed to help this condition are berries, garlic, onion, teas, broccoli, parsley, Soy foods, thyme, and legumes.

CBD Hemp Oil can provide the body the necessary nutrients and medicinal properties to fight against the bacteria in the stomach lining as well as the conditions associated with it. Traditional medicines for this disease use anti-acids like Rolaids, Maalox, Mylanta, etc., these medicines have a combination of calcium, aluminum, and magnesium that could cause diarrhea and constipation. CBD oil does not have many side effects that are associated with traditional medicine. The cannabinoid receptors present in the CBD oil have anti-inflammatory, analgesic, anti-emetic, anti-bacterial and anti-prokinetic.

The stated properties could lead to less inflammation in the inflamed area, less nausea and vomiting sensation, a higher sense of nerve-muscle coordination, and muscle relaxation. The studies done on the endocannabinoid system shows that the addition of natural and synthetic cannabinoids could help it become more in control of the gastrointestinal system. In the nerves surrounding the stomach lining, cannabinoid CB1 and endogenous cannabinoids are found that can contribute to the maintenance of a healthier stomach environment. These cannabinoids have been studied extensively; they show anti-inflammatory properties and inhibition in the gastrointestinal fluid secretion through clinical studies. Predominantly, the CBD, CBG, and THC (V) cannabinoids are responsible for the better health and reduction of the symptoms caused by gastritis. All of which are found abundantly in CBD-rich hemp oil.

PEPTIC ULCERS AND GASTRIC ULCERS

Peptic Ulcer develops on the lining of the small intestines that is known as the duodenum. If this ulcer is found in the stomach lining, then it would be known as a gastric ulcer. It is the erosion of the lining caused by acidity; it could be excruciating in some cases. The cause of erosion is a bacterium that lived in the stomach in an acidic environment. It causes inflammation by infecting the area; it cannot be removed by the natural immune system of the body.

The bacterium formation in the stomach area could cause an irregularity in the production of gastrin. Gastrin controls the gastric production acid in the body, increase the levels of the production of the acid could cause an erosion in the lining to cause ulcers. The decreased production of gastric can also produce other conditions such as hypo- or achlorhydria. Some consumables increase the risk of development of these ulcers by irritating the lining of the body, which can cause gastric acid to erode it. Drinking alcohol, using medicine like naproxen, ibuprofen, aspirin, and nonsteroidal anti-inflammatory can cause ulcers to develop. Smoking and radiation treatment are also considered to be one of the common causes of ulcers.

The symptoms associated with ulcers can be categorized as abdominal pain, hunger, thirst, nausea, pain or discomfort in the stomach area, chest pain, vomiting, fatigue, and weight loss. Most medicines either target some of these conditions or cause other side-effects on the body. CBD hemp oil can help alleviate many of the symptoms as well as reduce the chance of development of other ulcers.

The United States Institute of Medicine has also stated that CBD hemp oil would be very beneficial "For patients who suffer simultaneously from severe pain, nausea, and appetite loss, cannabinoid drugs might offer broad-spectrum relief not found in any other single medication." The cannabinoids found in CBD hemp oil can help the body relax while providing pain relieving properties. Moreover, the levels of the cannabinoid known as anandamide that is responsible for taking care of the gastrointestinal system can be raised higher through CBD hemp oil. This cannabinoid controls the gastrointestinal motility to offer anti-inflammatory properties; it also decreases the gastrointestinal fluid secretion causing the ulcers in the first place.

The cannabinoid receptors present in the CBD hemp bind together with the CBD receptors of the endocannabinoid system of the body. This can modulate the production of gastric acid production. It also has other properties such as increasing the nerve-coordination, providing relief to symptoms such as nausea and vomiting, providing pain relief properties in the targeted areas and reduced inflammation associated with the ulcers.

CROHN'S DISEASE

Crohn's disease is one of the most painful diseases associated with inflammation in the digestive tract. This disease is also known as the inflammatory bowel disease that causes many issues such as weight loss, diarrhea, fatigue, abdominal pains, and malnutrition. The inflammation caused by this disease can develop in different areas of the stomach for different people. The inflammation caused by the Crohn's disease could spread into other areas of the bowel to cause very painful and life-threatening complications.

The symptoms associated with this disease are caused by the irregularities in the small intestine and the colon. These symptoms gradually develop to cause painful spasms in the abdominal area, without any previous indications. The conditions that may appear due to this disease are abdominal pain, cramps, fever, diarrhea, fatigue, reduced appetite, weight loss, mouth sores, blood in the stools, inflammation in the joints, inflammation in the liver, and inflammation of the skin.

Recently, the cause of Crohn's disease was unknown; it was suspected that the condition developed due to stress and diet. The latest research on this condition has found out that, it develops due to the deficiency of the immune system and due to hereditary causes. The immune system may try to fight off the toxic products in the digestive tract and may attack the tissue linings of the stomach as well. The risk of developing this condition is increased by smoking and ingesting Nonsteroidal anti-inflammatory medications such as ibuprofen, naproxen, and others of the like.

This disease has many other complications that develop along with the primary symptoms. It may cause bowel obstruction due to the increase in thickness of the intestinal walls. It could also cause ulcers to develop in the digestive tract; the inflammation could also cause ulcers in the anal and mouth area. This inflammation could also cause other acute conditions such as Fistulas. The ulcer extends to develop a connection between other parts of the body such as skin or bladder. The pain associated with the inflammation could cause the individual to develop irregular eating habits that could lead to malnutrition.

The CBD cannabinoid plays an essential part in relieving many of the symptoms associated with Crohn's disease. This cannabinoid forms a connection with the CB1 and CB2 receptors in the endocannabinoid system of the body. This system controls many parts of the body such as the nervous system, brain, colon, and intestines. When this cannabinoid binds itself to the receptors in the body, it provides pain relieving, anti-inflammatory, anti-emetic responses in the body among others.

The regular use of CBD hemp oil also contributes to the increased production of white blood cells that could fight against inflammation and other illnesses. The National Institute of Health has also stated that CBD oil is very beneficial for gastrointestinal infections because of its multi-purpose properties.

Most of the pain and irregularities in the body are caused by weakness in the endocannabinoid system of the body. If it is out of sync with the rest of the systems in the body, then it may cause issues in the brain and the stomach. CBD hemp oil has concentrated CBD cannabinoid that acts as a "pick me up" for the endocannabinoid system to make stronger. This cannabinoid, among others, also connects with CB1 and CB2 receptors that move through the digestive tract to provide anti-inflammatory, analgesic, anti-emetic, anti-bacterial, and Anti-prokinetic properties.

EATING DISORDERS

Eating disorders could be caused by some issues such as upset stomach, pregnancy, cold. And other diseases. The loss of appetite is identified as a side effect that responsible for malnutrition in many diseases such as anxiety, depression, cancer, liver disease, dementia, and heart disease. Moreover, the loss of appetite is also attributed to other actions and such as recreational use of cocaine, heroin, morphine, antibiotics, and speed.

Cannabinoids present in the hemp oil can offer relief in many of the conditions mentioned above, which in turn raised the appetite of the individuals ingesting it regularly. The CB1 receptors, which are responsible for aiding many of the systems of the body through endocannabinoid system, are also responsible for producing strong feelings of hunger. It also reduces stress and anxiety that also helps people become more in tune with their health causing them to eat regularly. Some strains of hemp oil may contain a small ratio of THC cannabinoid, which is a proven appetite stimulant. Through the regular consumption of these strains, the individuals suffering from loss of appetite could be treated.

A recent study conducted by the American Psychological Association has stated that almost 30% of the adults participating in their survey had skipped their meal due to stress. While 67% of the adults that had skipped their attributed it to their loss of appetite. Other studies were done by the National Cancer Trust also show that the patients that had cancer or received radiation had a significant increase in their appetite by using CBD hemp oil regularly.

Moreover, the other effects of CBD hemp oil that are therapeutic can relieve the stress caused by various mental disorders to improve the overall health of the body. This could help individuals that suffer from stress-induced eating disorders like emotional eating or anorexia. The stronger endocannabinoid systems in the bodies of those that take CBD hemp oil could potentially have stronger health that could contribute to an increase in appetite.

USE OF CDB HEMP OIL FOR DIGESTIVE AND INFLAMMATORY DISEASES

CBD oil can be used to treat many digestive issues that cause inflammation and pain. Moreover, it could also act as an appetite stimulant to avoid malnutrition. The cannabinoid receptor moves on a molecular level in the systems of the body that is why it is best to ingest it in concentrations for best effects. The connections of the cannabinoids present in the body could help with the symptoms and pains associated with gastric ulcers, irritable bowel syndrome, diarrhea, Crohn's disease, and ulcers.

It is best to find a CBD hemp oil product that has been taken from naturally grown plants, with added chemicals it might become unsafe to use as a dietary supplement, especially for individuals with stomach issues. A pure CBD hemp oil has a mix of rich nutrients such as omega-3, omega-6, and proteins that are great as an additional supplement to the daily diet for individuals that have eating disorders. They also have anti-oxidant and vitamin-E constituents that beneficial for the overall health and environment of the digestive tract.

For immediate results and to relieve pain in issues such as gastritis and Crohn's, it is best to use CBD oil tinctures. The tinctures are usually available as oil drops. However, they may have different flavors to help with easier ingestion. They are a fast-acting CBD product that provides immediate effect through proper use. The Tincture should be held under the tongue for a few minutes so that the concentrate can be absorbed into the bloodstream through the tongue.

After a few minutes, it should be swallowed so the beneficial properties of the cannabinoids can help the stomach and the digest track through direct contact. The pure CBD hemp oil is formed through the concentrate of CBD that taken from the non-GMO hemp plant.

For the inflammation of joints and skin that appears with gastritis and Crohn's, it is best to use CBD hemp oil salves or crams. They can help hydrate the skin as well as reduce any inflammation of the skin immediately. The topical application of salves can also help with joint stiffness and dry spots that are an after effect of inflammation caused by digestive disorders.

Other forms of CBD oil that can help in the long-run and act as a supplementary addition to the daily routine is the CBD hemp oil capsules. These capsules are usually available in a bottle containing a monthly addition to the supplementary regiment. This addition will not only help with the digestive issues, but it will also act as a nutritional supplement. It is also available as a CBD hemp seed powder that can be added as an additive to other food items or drinks such as smoothies or juices. This is one of the most popular ways to consume CBD concentrate due to its convenience.

Recently, due to the boom in the popularity of CBD hemp oil, many companies have started infusing CBD oil into edible and chewable products that can act as a snack. There are many forms of CBD hemp oil edibles such as mini chocolate bars and gummies that are jam-packed with the nutrients found in the oil. These edibles can help individuals that have a sweet tooth as well other digestive issues find a more accessible alternative to get their fill of sweets. CBD honey and CBD peanut butter are also available for a quick an easier addition of CBD hemp oil into the breakfast regime.

CBD HEMP OIL AS ANTI-EPILEPTIC AND ANTI-SPASMODIC

The CBD cannabinoid shows a marked improvement in seizure disorders, unlike its THC counterpart. It has anticonvulsant properties that could attribute to the conditions caused by seizure disorders without any undesired effects such as being high as a side effect. Over the past years, CBD oil has been studied extensively; it has led the scientific world to believe that CBD-enrich extracts could be beneficial for young children. Other than the improvement in the seizures, it could also maintain other habits of behavior such as the sleeping pattern.

The connection of CBD hemp oil with the nervous system stems from the presence of the cannabinoid receptors such as the CB1 and CB2. The CB1 cannabinoid receptor is responsible for maintaining and controlling the central nervous system. Whereas, the CB2 receptor move through the molecular paths near the immune system. These receptors made way to the identification of other endogenous cannabinoids such as 2-arachidonoyl glycerol and 2-arachido-noylethanolamide/anandamide both of which play an important role in the regulation of neuronal firing and the synaptic transmission. By activating the growth of these receptors in the endocannabinoid system, the synaptic transmission could be inhibited to cause lesser epileptic episodes.

Research has also shown that different types of cannabinoids can provide anti-epileptic properties for different type's epilepsy or seizures. For example, the THC cannabinoid has many different and complex properties such as anti-inflammatory, cognitive, anticonvulsant effects, complex psychoactive effects, and appetite stimulant among others.

Whereas the CBD cannabinoid does not have the psychoactive effects, it possesses properties such as neuroprotection, anticonvulsant, immune-modulating, anticonvulsant, and antiemetic among others. Through preclinical studies, it has been concluded that CBD is an active anticonvulsant that helps with seizures brought on by electro-shock. It has also been effective against the focal seizures; it helps by protecting the pilocarpine models of the temporal lobe.

Another study done by the National Institute of Neurological Disorders and Stroke (NINDS) investigated the effects of CBD through their Epilepsy Therapy Screening Program. In which they experimented on mice to show that the dosage of the CBD concentrate may help with the reduction of seizure activity without any motor impairment.

The CB1 and CB2 receptors are also responsible for muscle relaxation to provide relief from muscle spasms. Most of the evidence that has been collected in its favor suggests that CBD hemp oil can reduce tremors and muscle spasm by regulation of the body and inhibits the neurotransmitter that causes spasms. The cannabinoids responsible for providing the properties that help with seizures and spasm are CBD, THC (V), CBN, and CBC (A). A point often overlooked is CBD hemp oil's multi-purpose abilities, it helps the endocannabinoid system, but it also helps the other system through its nutritional contents. Other properties may help with the after-effects of an epileptic attack, which is why this herbal remedy is often recommended to be added into the daily regiments of patients with epileptic disorders.

MUSCLE SPASMS

Muscle Spasms are caused when there are an involuntary contraction and tightening of the muscles; this causes pain and mobility issues in the associated joints. The frequency of the spastic attacks could be lessened through the use of CBD hemp oil. Most of the times muscle spasm is caused by extraneous work hours or dehydration, other times it may be a condition associated with other illnesses such as Multiple Sclerosis.

The spasm attack caused by MS is usually sudden movement or immediate change in the temperature of the atmosphere. The uncontrollable spastic attack leaves the muscle stiff and somewhat in pain, even after the attack is over. These attacks could appear throughout any limb muscle. However, it is commonly seen in the leg muscle.

Many studies have been implemented on the effect of CBD hemp oil on humans and animals. The CBD cannabinoid is responsible for reducing the spasticity and the tremors due to its connection with the CB1 and CB2 receptors found in the endocannabinoid system. For the spasms caused by MS, CBD hemp oil concentrate is recommended as it not only reduced the number of attacks but, it also offers relief in other conditions that are associated with it. After twelve months of use, there should be an evident decrease in the severity of the attack.

Research conducted on human participants also provided insight on the effectiveness of CBD hemp in a limited time frame. It was able to lessen the attacks within the use of three to four weeks. There has also been an improvement in the overall frequency of the attacks in patients with MS that had found no tradition treatment for the attacks.

The effects of CBD hemp oil has better effectiveness on young children that suffer from spasms because of various illnesses. The infantile children that suffered from spasms were given a regular dosage of CBD hemp. After a few weeks, there was a marked improvement in the frequency of the attacks. It also reduced the frequency of other destructive symptoms caused by the attacks such as West Syndrome.

The use of CBD hemp oil could also improve the quality of life as it has many beneficial effects due to its nutrient contents. The hemp oil provides the necessary fatty acids to the individuals ingesting it regularly. It could improve their overall health and cognitive abilities. Due to the multi-purpose properties of CBD hemp, it is often suggested to be added into the daily regiment for people with various issues and diseases.

EPILEPSY

Epilepsy can be a very difficult adversary to beat as it can cause individuals to live as a victim because it does not has any cure. The research done on CBD hemp oil stated that there is an impact on the epileptic patients that use CBD hemp oil. The CBD cannabinoid has many properties that could calm the internal systems of the body to provide relief.

The endocannabinoid system of the body has connections with the nervous system and the immune system, both of which play an important role in epileptic disorders. If there is a deficiency in the endocannabinoid system then the system that is associated with will be affected. Under the deficient condition, the stress on the system may cause seizure attacks and other complications associated with it.

The cannabinoid receptors found in the CDB hemp oil have been effective against the epileptic seizures caused by Lennox-Gastuat syndrome, Dravet syndrome, Doose Syndrome, Myoclonic absence, and idiopathic epilepsy among others. The decrease in the epileptic seizures with the use of CBD hemp oil is quite drastic in children that have seizure disorders. The estimated change in the frequency of seizures after four to one year of CBD Hemp oil use is 80% less than that of with traditional medicine,

Moreover, children that have epileptic disorders are often attributed to malnutrition because of their lack of appetite. The cannabinoids that are presented in the CBD hemp oil can act as an appetite stimulant to increase the overall condition of the patients. The hemp seed oil, in particular, contributes many nutritional benefits through regular use that can help with improved dietary conditions. This oil has 30% healthy fats that consist of essential fatty acids, alpha-linolenic acid (omega-3), and linoleic acid (omega-6). They are also an excellent source of protein that could provide 25% high-grade proteins. Their nutritional benefits are often seen in part with that of Chia seeds and Flaxseeds. The nutritional benefits could also help with the stiffness felt in the joints by the patients with the epileptic disorder. The balance of the omega-3 and omega-6 fatty acid contributes to the improvement in the mobility of joints. These essential fatty acids also help reduce itchiness and skin conditions that may develop due to inflammation caused by stiff joints.

Being a source of naturally obtained protein, it can help individuals get the essential amino acids needed to complete the protein deficiency in epileptic patients. The CBD hemp oil also has naturally occurring fiber in its constituents that could help with digestive issues occurring as a condition. It can help by giving valuable nutrients to the bacteria that create a healthy atmosphere in the stomach.

These nutritional benefits should be present in CBD hemp oil that has naturally obtained through non-GMO plants. As some CBD hemp oils may contain other additives and chemicals to improve the state and taste of the oil product. CBD hemp oil has many relaxing properties, as well as rich, healthy fats and proteins that could be used to relax the muscle in case of cluster seizures. This could bring pain-relieving properties to the areas that have become stiff during the attack, which could lower the frequency of the seizures by providing relaxation to the areas.

LENNOX-GASTAUT/DRAVIT/WEST SYNDROME

Lennox-Gastaut syndrome along with other infantile epileptic disorders such Dravit syndrome and West syndrome can be treated with the use of CBD hemp oil. These form of epileptic diseases are very rare that is why they don't have many traditional methods of treatment. However, there are some investigations using the endocannabinoid system to provide treatment for the seizures.

The experiment conducted with human participants used placebo treatment and CBD oil treatment on patients that had Lennox-Gastaut Syndrome. It was noted there was a decrease in the frequency of the epileptic seizures within the time frame of one month. The CBD oil was given to the patients daily with the dosage of 20mg/kg. This research showed that the effects of this disease could show improvement with regular use. However, the research is ongoing and may affect different individuals that have other complex conditions differently.

USE OF CDB HEMP OIL FOR SEIZURE AND SPASTIC DISORDERS

It is essential to find the right type of CBD hemp oil concentration for different kinds of issues. For seizure disorders, it is important to find a concentrate of CBD to get proper benefits. The premium quality CBD hemp oil in a bottle of 10Ml would contain 240mg of CBD, whereas, 25 mg of CBD as dosage would be effective in this case. The increased concentration of CBD cannabinoid will help with the easier transition between the receptors and the body. The CB1 receptor is responsible for the maintenance of the brain and the nervous system whereas, the CB2 is associated with the regulation of the immune system. Through the balance of these cannabinoids, a healthy body can be achieved with reduced frequency of any attacks related to these systems.

For seizures and other epileptic disorders, it is best to find a concentrated form of CBD hemp oil. There are many strains of CBD hemp oil that could be beneficial for this disorder. The strains are a mix of CBD and other cannabinoids that would help relax the body to reduce stress which in turn will reduce the frequency of the attacks.

Pure CBD hemp oil that does not have other cannabinoid is not harmful to the body; it may have different effects than a strain that is dedicated to reducing the frequency of seizures. The CBD oi can improve the overall health of the body and give it a therapeutic relief to reduce the stress. By taking an overdose of this pure concentrate will not have any lasting side-effects on the body, it is not dangerous or lethal.

The condition of the health of the body dramatically depends on the amount of CBD hemp oil one should ingest to get the required effects. It should always be remembered that natural remedies like CBD hemp oil often take some time to heal acute illnesses such as epileptic disorders. The condition's intensity also depends upon the amount of CBD hemp oil one should ingest.

- For mild disorders, a person with the weight of 31 to 60 lbs. should ingest 2 to 4 mg plus of CBD oil. A person with 61 to 100 lbs. Weight should ingest 4 to 6 mg plus of the oil. A person with the weight of 100 to 175 lbs. should ingest 6mg to 8mg of oil and a person of weight 175 to 250 lbs. should ingest 8 to 10mg of the oil regularly, granted that it is a pure concentrate or a specific strain dedicated for their illness.

- For medium disorders, a person with the weight of 31 to 60 lbs. Should ingest 4 to 8 mg plus of CBD oil. A person with 61 to 100 lbs. Weight should ingest 6 to 12 mg plus of the oil. A person with the weight of 100 to 175 lbs. should ingest 8mg to 18mg of oil and a person of weight 175 to 250 lbs. should ingest 12 to 20mg of the oil regularly, granted that it is a pure concentrate or a specific strain dedicated for their illness.

- For severe disorders, a person with the weight of 31 to 60 lbs. should ingest 12 to 18 mg plus of CBD oil. A person with 61 to 100 lbs. weight should ingest 18 to 24 mg plus of the oil. A person with the weight of 100 to 175 lbs. should ingest 24mg to 32mg of oil and a person of weight 175 to 250 lbs. should ingest 32 to 40mg of the oil regularly, granted that it is a pure concentrate or a specific strain dedicated for their illness.

This is a standard dose for people that need to start at one point. However, each person has a different constitution and may need different level dosages. It is always recommended for people that need to find the personalized dose that they start at the lowest dose recommended and increase it gradually depending upon the age, weight, and health condition.

CBD HEMP OIL AN ANTI-ISCHEMIC

CBD hemp oil has many constituents that have been identified to play an important role in healing various issues and disorders of the body. Most of these cannabinoids connect with cannabinoid receptors known as CB1 and CB2, which mainly exist in the molecular channels found in the peripheral and central nervous system. The CB2 receptors have also been identified in the nervous system, particularly, in the neutrophils and lymphocytes. There are other cannabinoid components present in the CBD hemp oil like cannabigerol (CBG) and cannabidivarin (CBDV) that have analgesic, anxiolytic, anti-cancer, and anti-inflammatory properties.

Moreover, these cannabinoids connect with different receptors found in the endocannabinoid system to provide anticonvulsant, anxiolytic, and anti-rheumatoid arthritis properties. Furthermore, the CBD cannabinoid has been shown to have protective properties against beta-amyloid peptide and N-methyl-D-aspartate that are known to cause ischemic injuries.

A study conducted by Hampson in 1998 also showed that the CBD cannabinoid could act as a powerful anti-oxidant. It was considered to be fast acting and provided more efficacy than the THC constituent. CBD cannabinoid exhibited far stronger antioxidant properties that could potentially protect against hippocampal-entorhinal-cortical neurodegeneration. This property attributed its effects as a therapeutic drug that could act as a potent anti-oxidant that can be used after an ischemic stroke because t often causes oxidant disorder.

 Another comparative study that was done in 1974 also demonstrated that CBD hemp oil could be an effective anxiolytic drug. It activated those receptors in the forebrain region that were responsible for better locomotor functions and improved cognitive activities. Through this data, it could be concluded that CBD hemp oil may also significantly improve the functional and cognitive impairment caused by cerebral ischemia.

On the other hand, THC constituents were found to cause various conditions such as hypoactivity and catalepsy in individuals that repeatedly took its concentrate. CBD did not cause these issues nor did it cause ant development of a tolerance for cerebroprotective effects. Even after using CBD hemp pol regularly for two weeks, there were no side effects; rather it caused neuroprotective effects in individual using it.

CBD hemp oil also has powerful anti-inflammatory properties that could help in the ischemic treatment.

It could help with the post-ischemic injuries that are caused by ischemic strokes. This is due to its ability to reduce and inhibit the plasma high-mobility from the damaged and dying cells, which in turn lowers the risk of heart attacks.

CARDIOVASCULAR DISEASES

Cardiovascular diseases such as Cardiac Ischemia or Myocardial ischemia is caused when the blood flow to the heart is reduced; it causes the heart to receive less blood. The reduced blood flow is attributed to the blockage of the arteries of the heart. Multiple attacks of this disease may be fatal because it severely damages the heart muscle as well as its ability to pump blood. It may also cause the heart to develop irregular rhythm causing conditions such as nausea and heart palpitations. The treatment for this disease includes improving the blood flow to the muscles of the heart. The medication mostly focuses on opening the blocked pathway in the arteries; it can also cause the individuals to receive bypass surgery.

The symptoms associated with cardiac ischemia are typically felt on the left side of the body, this pain is known as angina pectoris. Other symptoms for women of patients that have diabetic issues are neck or jaw pain, pain in the arm or shoulder, breathing issues during activities, abnormal heartbeat, sweating, nausea, fatigue, and vomiting are also conditions that are associated with this disease. Other conditions that develop due to atherosclerosis are coronary artery disease, heart failure, heart arrhythmia, cardiomyopathy, atrial fibrillation, cardiac arrest, endocarditis, dyslipidemia, and myocarditis.

The cause of the blocked arteries can be a slow process; it could develop due to several causes. Coronary artery disease is one of the causes for the blockage in the arteries that cause cardiac ischemia. With this disease, the plaque that is built in the arteries is mostly due to the cholesterol build up. Atherosclerosis clogs the arteries with plaque built up from cholesterol; it is also one of the leading causes that develop myocardial ischemic diseases.

The plaque in the arteries of the heart can also build up due to a blood clot that appears due to an artery rupture. This rupture could appear due to Atherosclerosis. The blood clot may build up to cause a severe and acute heart attack as a myocardial ischemic attack.

Moreover, this blood clot may pass through the heart arteries to flow into other parts of the body to cause nerve damage, albeit, this only happens rarely. The other cause of cardiac ischemia may be coronary artery spasm, which is the tightening of the muscles of the artery wall. It could cause a minor blood flow irregularity. An increased amount of spasms may cause the arteries to become blocked, which would further instigate myocardial ischemia.

This condition can be irritated by smoking as it may damage the arteries, which would cause them to collect cholesterol and other substances that could cause a blockage. It also increases the risk of blood clots. Patients that suffer from diabetic disorders are also at risk of developing myocardial diseases. High cholesterol and high blood pressure can damage the coronary arteries. The increased cholesterol levels are associated with a diet high in cholesterol and saturated fats. Obesity can also cause the walls of the arteries to become thicker and reduce the amount of blood flow to the heart.

CBD hemp oil brings the risk of developing any of these issues due to its multipurpose properties. The cannabinoid receptors play an important part in reducing the conditions associated with cardiac ischemia. The receptors activate the body's naturally occurring healing properties through their cannabinoids. One of these cannabinoids is CBD, whose deficiency or irregularity may cause many conditions associated with cardiac ischemia to develop.

The regular use of CBD hemp oil can relax the arterial walls of the heart. By relaxing the overall arteries connected to the heart, it can reduce the risk of inflammation and clotting. Also, it is also very effective against the metabolic issues that are often seen as a risk for heart patients. Concentrate of CBD hemp oil has also reduced the permeability of the heart arteries. Inflammation of the arteries due to the development of plaque can also become a cause of tissue damage surrounding the heart. This inflammation could cut down the amount of blood flow moving through the arteries.

CBD hemp being a powerful anti-inflammatory drug offer anti-inflammatory properties along with anti-oxidant properties. The regular use of this oil could reduce the damage already caused by previous heart attacks because of its properties. It reduces the production of endotoxin that causes inflammatory conditions in the arteries of the heart. By inhibiting the production of the pro-inflammatory cytokines known as toxins, the CBD can lower the risk of a potential heart attack caused by cardiac ischemia.

CBD has also been studied to show a reduction of the plaque in the arteries. This could reduce the risk of development of heart and cardiovascular diseases. The studies done on CBD show that it reduces the ability of the plaque to adhere to the arterial walls. This could solve the problem of the plaque buildup in the arterial walls causing other complications.

Overall, the use of CBD hemp oil would also reduce inflammation and inhibit the pro-inflammatory cytokines, it also repairs the damaged tissues of the heart and reduced the plaque build-up in the arterial walls. The regular use of CBD hemp oil could help patients struggling with heart-related cardiovascular diseases.

CONGENITAL HEART DEFECT

This heart disease is often mixed up with cardiovascular diseases since both of them affect the blood vessels and the heart. However, it should be noted that Congenital Heart Defect is present at birth and are identified as birth-defects. There are many different types of Congenital Heart Defects that could cause many complications to little or no complications. The complexity of this disease may cause the infant to live with medicinal help all their life. This disease could be associated with an abnormality in the chromosomes, genetic, medications during pregnancy, and drug abuse during pregnancy among others.

CBD hemp oil can act as a potent vasorelaxant, meaning it could relax the arteries of the heart. The reduced tension in these arteries could decrease the risk of cardiovascular conditions associated with it. A review conducted on the cardiovascular system by Christopher P Stanley et al. also stated that

"Cannabidiol (CBD) has beneficial effects in disorders as wide-ranging as diabetes, Huntington's disease, cancer, and colitis. Accumulating evidence now also suggests that CBD is beneficial in the cardiovascular system." The CBD can directly isolate the issues in the arteries and could regulate the tension in the walls through its vasorelaxation properties. Another one of its most beneficial properties is its anti-oxidant and anti-inflammatory properties that could help patients that are at risk of developing acute or severe heart conditions.

In contrast to the therapeutic benefits of this oil, there many nutritional benefits for people that struggle with heart diseases. Hemp seed oil has the nutritional contents that could fight against inflammation. It has a significant amount of gamma linoleic acid, otherwise known as the omega-6 acid that helps fight inflammation and boost the immunity of the body. These nutritional components of the hemp oil promote the production of hormone-like chemicals known as prostaglandins that reduce inflammation in all parts of the body.

CBD hemp oil is also an excellent natural source of protein, which makes it develop anti-inflammatory properties. These properties of hemp can reduce inflammation in the heart muscles as well relieve the arthritic symptoms of the body. This oil is abundant in bioactive compounds that lower the blood cholesterol levels to protect the cardiovascular muscle and tissues. The ratio of omega-3 and omega-6 fatty acids is 1:3, which is considered to ideal for health. The maintenance of an ideal dosage of these fatty acids could be very beneficial for the health of the heart and relating tissues.

The research conducted on hemp seed oil also states that the absorption of cholesterol in the body could be reduced with regular use. Another study also dictates that by taking 30ml of hemp seed oil every day can help the body absorb less harmful cholesterol, which can improve the overall health of the heart. The essential fatty acids like omega-3 and omega-6 can reduce the absorption of harmful fatty acids into the body, which in turn enhances and promotes the cardiovascular health.

Hemp seed oil also maintains the nutritional balance of the body by providing it the necessary fatty acids too work in optimum order, this supplementary addition to the diet could reduce the overall stress on the body, which will lower the chance of any complications to arise in various illnesses.

 Diabetes could cause inflammation in heart arteries because of all the complications associated with it, it could cause the patient to develop cardiovascular diseases, or it could irritate the heart condition of congenital heart defect of patients.

Hemp seed oil can reduce the risk of developing diabetes as it maintains a healthy glucose level in the body and gives a boost to the endocannabinoid system to help develop regular eating patterns. The fatty acid content of CBD oil can also fight against the inflammation caused in other regions as well; it could inhibit the growth of cancer in the brain and breast through regular use. Weak immunity may cause the patient with a congenital heart defect to develop other complications and fall quickly. Through the use of proper omega-3 fats and GLA, the immune system could be brought to a better condition. These fatty acids are found in hemp seed oil, they boost the immunity of weakened patients and prevent diseases of all kind.

USE OF CDB HEMP OIL FOR HEART DISEASES

Heart diseases, for the most part, occur when there is a buildup of plaque in the artery walls that is why there is a need of control of the cholesterol levels, inflammation, blocked arteries, and so forth. CBD hemp seed oil has many properties that could help patients with heart disease find management system. The CBD hemp oil has two system through which it could help patients with heart disease. The hemp oil could help the patient have lower cholesterol levels and have the necessary nutrients to develop a cardiovascular system.

The CBD concentrate in the CBD hemp oil could offer help to the endocannabinoid system by presenting cannabinoids that connect with the cannabinoid receptors in the body to offer many properties. Some of the properties that the cannabinoids offer to the endocannabinoid system are anti-inflammation, ant-ischemia, analgesic, anti-epileptic, and neuroprotective among many other properties.

Hempseed oil has many high levels of essential amino acids, particularly the amino acid arginine that is responsible for the control of the hemostasis of the body. This could lower the risk of damaging the blood vessels of the body to reduce any risk of a heart attack. The International Study of Macro-Micronutrients and Blood Pressure also concluded that the intake of hemp seed oil significantly decreased the blood pressure of the participants. Moreover, those participants that had hypertension noted that they felt a soothing sensation by using hemp seed oil regularly. A controlled study of patients with coronary heart disease showed that there was a 5% reduction in the risk of a heart attack.

There is no risk of using CBD hemp oil for heart patient. However, it is necessary for them to take the oil in proportion to their age, weight, and nature of the disease. Patients of heart should take CBD hemp oil in the form of edibles or pills as it is necessary for them that the contents of the oil remain in their body to help with the various complications associated with their particular disease.

If there is an associated inflammation and stiffness in the body after an attack, then the CBD hemp topical treatment is advised. As the topical treatment is fast acting and could provide relief for pain as well as the inflammation in the joint after an ischemic attack.

CBD HEMP OIL AS AN ANTIFUNGAL

Fungus, unlike, bacteria have a DNA-containing nucleus, they act more like the living cells of the human body. For this reason, it is quite hard to fight off fungal infections that are often seen on the skin tissue of the body. Most of the common and traditional treatment for the fungal infections are not easy to find because of their same structural similarities. Like humans need nutrients, fungi need a compound known as ergosterol to maintain the structure and strength of their walls.

The medicine found for the treatment of these infections reduced the production of ergosterol, which prevents the fungi to grow and gradually kills it. Every cannabinoid that is found in the CBD hemp oil is a powerful anti-inflammatory and has other properties that deal with many other mild to serious issues such reducing the growth of cancer cells and the increase of growth of brain cells.

The best properties of CBD hemp oil that are known to medically valuable stem from the antimicrobial factors in the cannabinoids such as CBD, CBC, and CBD. The most important constituent of CBD hemp oil that has powerful antifungal abilities is CBC (A). Moreover, turpentine that is also found in abundance in this oil is a powerful anti-fungal. Terpenes are compounds that are found in all species of plants; they are responsible for the smells associated with each plant. They are very effective homeopathic agents and can relieve the symptoms of pain, anxiety, and inflammation. Terpenes and cannabinoids have a common precursor, which attributes to their binding ability and effectiveness against various issues.

Focusing more on the effectiveness of the cannabinoid, it is assuredly said that the CBD and CBG have more effectiveness against fungal infections than the CBD cannabinoid, which is considered to have mild antifungal effects. The studies done on the antifungal properties of CBD hemp oil has claimed that the CBG and CBD cannabinoids are very effective for the inhibition of onychomycosis, which as widespread infection found in humans.

The rate of eradication of the onychomycosis is far greater than the pharmaceutical antifungals that are commonly found in medicine containing sulconazole and cyclopiroxolamine. The terpene having the composition of caryophyllene oxide was also found to be effective for inhibiting the growth of fungal infections.

Going further into detail, the cannabinoids consist of hydroxyl groups, where each oxygen atom is attached with a single hydrogen atom. OH, the group is known to be very antioxidant and reactive. When in touch with ergosterol compound that the fungi thrive with, it completely overtakes and oxidizes it, making the growth of further ergosterol compound impossible.

ATHLETE'S FOOT/ RINGWORM/ JOCK ITCH

Most of the fungal infections grow in damp and humid environments that give them a perfectly warm and moist atmosphere where they can thrive. Athlete's foot is commonly found in the soft part in-between the toes. This fungal infection develops in people that wear sports shoes and closed shoes often, where the sweat accumulates.

This type of fungal infection often occurs in warm and humid climates during summer and spring months. The symptoms associated with this illness are itchiness in the area, scaling or peeling away of the skin, blister, stinging, and burning sensation on the skin. This type of fungal infection could be easily dealt with topical ointments.

Jock itch occurs with the same fungi overgrowth as the athlete's foot; it usually occurs in the inner thigh and the groin area. It could cause the area to become irritated, inflamed, or chaffed. Ringworm, another by-product of the same fungi infection as the athlete's foot. It grows on the dead skin cells near the hair, nails, and other skin parts.

It is identified by a red patch that forms in a ring-like pattern that surrounds scaly or patchy skin. These type of infections are contagious and be transmitted through skin contact or by petting animals that have this infection. This infection can also be improved by keeping the area dry, so the environment becomes inhabitable for further growth of the fungus.

CBD hemp oil can be used to address these areas for relief and removal of the infection. Being a fungal herb, it can fight against the growth of the fungal infection by slowing its structural growth. It can be used as a topical treatment to ward off the resistant fungal infections that won't go away with the preventive measures.

YEAST INFECTION

Yeast infection is one of the most common infections that are associated with women; it is caused by the increased growth of Candida albicans, which causes candida infections. This growth in the candida fungi might be due to an imbalance of the naturally present yeast and bacteria in the body because of the use of antibiotic or hormone imbalance; it could also be due to stress or poor eating habits. The symptoms that are associated with this condition are itching, inflammation of the area, soreness, and redness, and other such complications.

To eliminate the imbalance created by the causes mentioned above it is important to eat a properly balanced meal. Foods such as processed sugar, soy products, aged cheese, fruits, vinegar, and carbohydrates such as grains, pasta, cereal, and bread should be avoided. By eliminating these food items, the environment that made the infection thrive could be removed. However, to get the nutrients that were lost by removal of the above mention food items other high-quality food items should be added. These food items could be milk yogurt, healthy fats like in avocado, hemp oil, coconut oil, nuts, seeds, and vegetable oils such as pumpkin, hemp, flax, and virgin olive oil.

In light of the above mention facts, it can be said that CBD hemp oil is a naturally powerful supplement for the people susceptible to yeast infections. The hemp oil has the dietary compounds that could help with various complications that arise with this infection. The CBD helps with the inflammation and itchiness, whereas, the hemp provides the nutritional benefits. The fatty acids present in the hemp oil could eliminate the infection by making the environment unfriendly for further growth of an infection.

USE OF CBD HEMP OIL FOR FUNGAL INFECTIONS

Skin infections such as fungal infection could be due to a dietary imbalance and unsanitary conditions of the skin. It is important for the body to get the necessary nutrients to fight off bad bacterium and unwanted fungal infections. One of the most common preventatives for fungal infections is to keep up with the hygiene of the body. It is important the body maintains its normal state to get in the best hygienic shape. To prevent fungal infections, it is important that you bath regularly to keep the area clean and the environment inhabitable for the fungi. Other important preventative is to take in the necessary nutrients to avoid weakening the skin, which would make it susceptible to infections.

CBD hemp oil can be applied topically to infections such as athlete's foot and ringworm that are present in open areas. This could help by inhibiting the growth of the bacteria and making the skin less irritated. As it is a powerful anti-inflammatory drug, it can help tone down the redness associated with the infected area. The CBD cannabinoid will also give relief for any burning and itching sensation that is felt by the fungal infection as it has analgesic properties. CBD hemp oil can be easily found as a topical treatment in the form of balms and creams that could be applied in the affected areas.

Further growth of these infections could be reduced by using CBD hemp oil skin and hair products such CBD shampoos or body washes that could keep the area clean and have the anti-fungal effects to fight off infections. The hemp oil can be taken as an edible or as a liquid through different products available in the market. CBD oil is available as candies, concentrated liquid, and tinctures. However, for fungal infection, it is often advised that it should be taken as a pill.

Through pill CBD hemp oil products, the effects of the constituents should be more effective and long-lasting.

Moreover, the hemp oil could help alleviate the imbalance of diet that had previously caused the skin infection. CBD hemp oil products should be taken by the weight of the body, the age, and health of the individual. It does not have any fatal effects if taken in excess. However, there may be slight discomfort if the dosage is not up to the mark. Clinically, it has been recommended to take at least two pills of CBD hemp oil to get the benefits properly. It could help with various other conditions as well as the skin infections of the body.

CHAPTER FOUR - PSYCHOLOGICAL BENEFITS OF CBD HEMP OIL

Mental health has been dealt with various modes of modern pharmaceuticals. Specific medication has been made to deal with mental health issues such as panic attacks, anxiety, depression, and so forth. Each one of these health disorders has a complex background that cannot be dealt with just one medication. The severity of the condition also changes a lot in the medication that would be offered for it. This complexity of mental health disorders causes unwanted effects through traditional modes of medication; it could even further destabilize the mental health issue.

Recently, CBD cannabinoid has been researched as a better alternative than the modern pharmaceuticals as it has many properties that could naturally balance the mental health of individuals. Moreover, there are no side effects that have been associated with the use of CBD hemp oil for the treatment of mental health issues. The connection between the endocannabinoid system and these cannabinoids forms a connection that could potentially help with various mental health disorders. They could help manage other complications that exist with mental health issues such as pain, mood, and appetite imbalance.

CBD cannabinoid creates a balance of the cannabinoids with the endocannabinoid system to help regulate various other systems that are controlled by it. The cannabinoids associated with providing balanced mental health are CBN and CBD. Both of which help the body keep an active state of mind by giving proper sleeping routine and the necessary chemicals to keep happy and healthy.

By maintaining a stable and balance endocannabinoid system, the body can achieve the state of healthy homeostasis. An imbalance in the endocannabinoid system could cause the neurotransmitters to behave erratically or irregularly, which could cause a change in the production and absorption of the serotonin.

A balanced endocannabinoid system can control the neurotransmitters that are responsible for the communication between the brain cells. The different cannabinoids that are found in the CBD hemp oil can effects differently for different illnesses. CBD hemp oil has an impressive psychological effect on the mental health of the user with imposing any psychoactive side-effects, unlike marijuana or cannabis. The use of CBD hemp oil has been also associated with the treatment of substance abuse and drug dependency disorders. It could treat the individuals that suffer from addiction disorders from the addictive substance such as alcohol or drugs. It has been noted that CBD oil can become a proper management system to reduce the craving that is felt by the cigarette smoking excess drinking of alcohol.

CBD can reduce the craving associated with the various addictive by acting as a shield for the brain, so it does not feel any irregularities in its system. This is done by maintaining a balance with the endocannabinoid system of the body. His system can control the emotional aftereffects of the addictive as well as the cravings that are associated with it.

That is why, now endocannabinoid system is considered as one of the most important systems of the body, which often overlooked. This system can be made stronger by giving it the necessary components such as cannabinoids that are balanced. These cannabinoids are present in the CBD hemp oil, and by regular use of this oil, the endocannabinoid system could balance to maintain a healthy mind and body.

CBD HEMP OIL AS ANTI-ANXIOLYTIC

Some clinical researchers have been implemented on CBD hemp oil and its effects as anti-anxiolytic. The CBD cannabinoid can work with the CB1 receptor of the body's endocannabinoid system. These receptors work on molecular levels as proteins to boot the chemical signals of various systems so they can work better and quickly respond. In the same way, these receptors can help with the production of serotonin. Serotonin plays a very important part in making sure that the individual has stable mental health. Decreased production of serotonin can cause many mental health complications such as anxiety and depression.

The traditional treatment associated with such mental issues is Prozac or Zoloft that are modified to offer balance in the individual mental state. National

Institute on Drug Abuse conducted a study of CBD on animals for generalized anxiety disorders, the conclusion of this study led to believe that CBD can improve many behavioral signs that are associated with anxiety disorders such as increased heart rate. Other studies also confirmed that it has many beneficial properties that could help many symptoms associated with post-traumatic stress disorder (PTSD) and social anxiety disorder (SAD).

A report in *Journal of Psychopharmacology* also studied the effects of CBD on patients with social anxiety disorders. The research gave half the participants 400 milligrams of CBD oil oral dose, while the others were given a placebo pill. The participants that received the CBD dose had a significant decrease in their anxiety levels.

Long-term effects of this herb have not been studied. However, other short clinical studies have shown positive re-enforcement in the department that is pro-CBD hemp oil for mental health issues. Another clinical study conducted by Scott Shannon, an assistant clinical professor of Psychiatry at the University Of Colorado School Of Medicine in Fort

Collins, also concluded that CBD could contribute to the behavioral issues and impaired mental health. This study presented a girl with PTSD symptoms as well other mental complicated problems like insomnia and anxiety.

To treat her various issues, CBD hemp oil was also added as a potential treatment that eventually showed positive results. The girl was given CBD concentrate for two months through which her anxiety and insomnia were fixed. They also used a high dosage of CBD hemp oil spray for the treatment of her anxiety during her attacks. It was noted that after five months of CBD use, there was a gradual decrease in the overall mental health issues that the girl was exhibiting.

Through research, it was concluded that CBD hemp oil could be an effective treatment for anxiety disorders and insomnia as well as PTSD, whose attacks were largely reduced in frequency. Hemp also hemp the participant receives the necessary nutrients as well as medication to become less anxious and to display normal behavior. It was concluded that the cannabinoid such as CBD and CBN could aid patients with insomnia and anxiety disorder through regular use.

ANXIETY DISORDERS

A large population of individuals suffers from an anxiety-related disorder. For some of the patients, there is not much improvement in their issues by using the traditional medicine. Moreover, the drugs responsible for improving the anxiety disorders such as Valium and Xanax are also very addictive. It is a harsh slope where one the solution of one issue leads to the development of other problems. The properties of CBD hemp oil are one of the most popular alternatives as a natural remedy for anxiety disorders. These disorders can be easily dealt with the use of CBD as it is non-addictive and does not have any side effects.

A tremendous amount of research has been on the properties of CBD hemp oil, many of which concluded that CBD hemp oil could be taken as an anti-anxiety herb. It could treat some anxiety-related disorders such as Panic disorder, Generalized Anxiety Disorder (GAD), Post-Traumatic Stress Disorder (PTSD),

Social phobia, Obsessive Compulsive Disorder (OCD), and Mild to moderate depression.

The CBD hemp oil has cannabinoids that target the production of a subtype of serotonin receptor known as 5-HT1A. Through the regulation of 5-HT1A, the anxiety disorders such as depression and anxiety could be treated. The serotonin system of the body is often a target of the target companies so it that aim to develop better production of the serotonin. They work by blocking absorption of the already existing serotonin to trick the brain to produce more in the synaptic space. Through this increased production of serotonin, there is a boost in the anxiety disorders.

Another study conducted by Spanish researchers has also stated that CBD can heighten the power of serotonin receptors that allow the treatment of other complications, which could not be solved by traditional medicine. The Spanish researchers stated that "The fast onset of antidepressant action of CBD and the simultaneous anxiolytic (anti-anxiety) effect would solve some of the main limitations of current antidepressant therapies." Another area of the brain that plays an important role in balancing the health of the brain is hippocampus.

Individuals with smaller hippocampus are often seen to be affected by anxiety disorders, the treatment for this issue is through the production of new neurons known as neurogenesis. CBD hemp oil can increase the production and regeneration rate of these neurons in the hippocampus through regular use.

DEPRESSION

Depression is one of the most common mental health disorder in the world; it could cause serious issues in the behavior of the people diagnosed with it. It causes the individual diagnosed with this ailment to become physically and emotionally distressed; it could cause many problems in the home and work life of the individual. Some of the symptoms that are associated with depressions are that the individual loses interest in their hobbies, there is a change in their appetite, they feel tired or fatigue all the time, their sleeping habits are disturbed as well, they also have negative thoughts, and trouble is making decisions in their life.

The cause of depression stems from many circumstances, it could be due to the imbalance in the biochemistry of the body, depression also runs in the family through genetics, and the environmental exposure to certain attitudes and neglect could also cause depression in the individual. There are many types of depressive disorders such as persistent depressive disorder; this disorder is also known as dysthymia. It could last a lifetime and cause mild to severe depressive episodes in the life of the individual suffering from it.

Another type of disorder that common in females is postpartum depression, it is also called baby blues at times. This name originates due to the anxiety and mild depression that the women feel after giving birth. This type of depression could change into severe depression and may change later into a mild form of depression. It causes a lot of stress on new mothers that have given birth, taking care of themselves and the baby along with this type of depression is very difficult.

Seasonal anxiety disorder is also a type of anxiety and depressive disorder. The causes of this depression might be receiving less sunlight; it is commonly associated with the winter season. It could also change the behaviors of the patients by imposing irregular sleeping habits, weight gain, and withdrawal. Another type of depressive disorder that is associated with irregular episodes is the Bipolar disorder; it is also known as bipolar depression. This type of depressive disorder causes the individual to feel episodes of high and low, where they may behave erratically or in a euphoric manner. This type of disorder can also develop into a mild form of hypomania.

CBD hemp oil has many strains that have different concentration of the cannabinoids that are present in it. The CBD oil that is a concentrate of CBD cannabinoid can have potent abilities as a mood stabilizer. It has been subscribed to many individuals that have been given Lamictal (pharmaceutical medicine for bipolar disorders), so they can have mood stabilization as well as a natural medicine for the seizures associated with it. The CBD properties have been found to be extremely similar to that of this pharmaceutical medicine.

The properties associated with CBD hemp also show improvement in the mood of the individuals by taking the edge off without causing any highness. Many individuals with depressive disorders that could be treated with modern medicine have started using CBD hemp oil as an alternative; it does not have any side effects that are long-lasting or severe. It has proved to be a powered ant depressive if taken in high dosages for a long term.

ANXIETY AND PANIC ATTACKS

Panic disorders are caused in individuals that struggle with anxiety disorders. This disorder is developed because of the overwhelming fear and anxiety that felt by the individual; it may lead to an increase in the frequency of the panic attacks. They are usually categorized as an intense wave of anxiety that causes immobility and many other complications. There are many symptoms that are associated with panic attacks such as hyperventilation, heart palpitations, discomfort, chest pain, hot or cold flashes, feeling detached from your surroundings, feeling light-headed, dizzy, or faint, choking feeling, trembling, numbness, tingling sensations, fear of going crazy, dying, or losing control, sweating, and nausea.

Panic attacks often occur on their own time and do not have a definite cause; they could be avoided by using some self-help techniques. Anxiety attacks or panic disorders could be caused by the feeling distress and fear of the unknown, it could benefits individuals by learning about their disorders, and the fight or flight response that is associated with it. Panic attacks could also be provoked through smoking, drinking in excess, and through caffeinated drinks. Some medications such as diet pills could also have stimulants that could cause heightened anxiety in individuals.

Hyperventilation is one of the most commonly associated complications with panic attacks; it could cause tightness and lightheadedness in the chest during the attacks. This symptom can be handled through deep breathing technique that could relieve other symptoms of the panic attack as well. Through the controlled breathing, the attention is diverted that limits the body to be in an active state for other mild issues connected with panic disorders.

Symptoms of anxiety induced panic disorders could also be considerably lowered by maintaining a healthy body through regular exercise. Exercise has been known as a natural anxiety reliever. Simple exercises such as walking, running, and jumping could help the body maintain a healthy state.

Panic disorders are experienced in an intense situation of anxiety that could be caused in individuals suffering from many other anxiety-related disorders such as Generalized Anxiety Disorder (GAD), Obsessive-Compulsive Disorder (OCD), and Post-Traumatic Stress Disorder (PTSD). The generalized anxiety disorder is categorized as the anxiety that felt by the disturbance in the life of individuals that have anxiety issues. It could cause individuals to feel anxiety with small changes or irregular environmental conditions. It may be caused by the disturbance in the daily routine or during other stress-inducing routines.

Panic disorders are also caused in individuals suffering from obsessive-compulsive disorder, where individuals feel the need to keep up with a lifestyle choice or routine. Any change in the choice or routine could cause them to lose control of their behavior and obsess over the irregularity. This could cause anxiety and panic attacks during the irregular situations.

Another type of anxiety that could cause panic attacks is the social anxiety disorder, this disorder could affect individual to behave erratically in social situations. Those people that are diagnosed with this disorder tend to move away from social situations as it may cause them anxiety.

Post-Traumatic Stress Disorder (PTSD) is caused in individuals that have experienced traumatic situations that could be life-threatening or something of the likes. This type of disorder can last a long time and cause other mental health issues to arise as well. CBD hemp oil has many cannabinoids that could help with anxiety and panic disorders.

THC and CBD both have very potent anti-anxiety properties. However, THC could cause other psychotic side effects with use. CBD, on the other hand, can remarkably treat many issues related to panic disorder without any mental health side effects. CBD hemp oil is a natural remedy for anxiety that instigates many disorders caused in individuals. It has also used as an anxiety drug by individuals that suffer from social anxiety disorders during situations such as public speaking or speech.

A number of researchers from the University of São Paulo, Ribeirão Preto also concluded that anxiety levels could be decreased in individuals that suffered from mild anxiety disorder through regular use of concentrated CBD hemp oil. This research studied the effects of CBD hemp oil on patients suffering from generalized anxiety disorders through a small double-blind study. There was a significant decrease in the anxiety levels of the individuals taking regular dosage of CBD hemp oil. A brain scan of the participants was also taken by the researchers; it also concluded that there was a change in the cerebral blood flow due to the anti-anxiety properties of CBD hemp oil.

Another study conducted by some professional researchers from the National Institute for Translational Medicine, School of Pharmaceutical Sciences of Ribeirão Preto, Institute of Neurosciences, University of Southern Santa Catarina, and School of Pharmaceutical Sciences of Ribeirão Preto also stated that CBD could help individuals with anxiety disorders during social situations.

This research was conducted on individuals that suffered from social anxiety disorders that had to publically speak in numerous situations. The participants reported a significant decrease in the anxiety, which later was noted to be because of lower blood pressure and heart rate. The researchers stated on that *"[CBD] significantly reduced anxiety, cognitive impairment, and discomfort in their speech performance, whereas the placebo group experienced "higher anxiety, cognitive impairment, [and] discomfort,"* which could conclude that CBD hemp oil can act as an anti-anxiety medicine for individuals that suffer from anxiety-related disorders.

SUBSTANCE ABUSE AND DEPENDENCY DISORDER

Many individuals sufferer from addiction-related disorder, they may be addicted to drugs or alcohol. These drugs are usually taken because the individual feels helpless in stress-inducing situations. To find relief from this situation, many individuals indulge in activities such as substance abuse. Through the regular use of these drugs and drinking, they could become dependent. Their inherent reaction to a stressful situation could be turning to drink or taking drugs.

This addiction could cause issues in the social life of the individuals as well as their personal lives. Family relations could become very weak due to the isolation induced by addiction. Further appearance in a social situation could cause anxiety in an individual that would cause them to backtrack and use drugs to put distance between themselves and the world.

Substance abuse and addiction could be caused in young individuals, adults, or senior adults due to many issues such as erratic routine, stress from the job, family issues, eating disorders, or mild to moderate anxiety disorders. Where addiction has been categorized by American Society of Disease Medicine as an individual's *"inability to consistently abstain, impairment in behavioral control, craving, diminished recognition of significant problems with one's behaviors and interpersonal relationships, and dysfunctional emotional response. Like other chronic diseases, addiction often involves cycles of relapse and remission. Without treatment or engagement in*

*recovery activities, addiction is progressive and can
result in disability or premature death.*"

This disease could be managed by developing proper behaviors of life and balanced mental health. CBD hemp oil has the cannabinoids that could moderate the behavior of the individuals through a wide range of anti-anxiety and mood-regulating abilities. High dosage of CBD hemp oil can also curb smoking and alcohol addiction in individuals. Through the study done by the Clinical Psychopharmacology Unit at University College London, it was concluded that CBD hemp significantly reduced the smoking behaviors of the individuals in a placebo pill clinical test.

There was a 40% decrease in the number of cigarettes smoked by individuals that were given CBD hemp oil. The decrease in smoking was due to the CBD hemp oil's reinforcement abilities, where it could stimulate the neurons and repaired them from being desensitized. The neurons of the brain are desensitized by smoking cigarettes; this could bring mild euphoric feeling. However, it could cause other long-term effects such as insomnia, irritability, and anxiety.

CBD hemp oil has cannabinoid constituents that can have neuroprotective abilities, which can help individuals that drink in excess. Drinking excess alcohol could cause neurodegeneration, where the neurons in our brain are slowly killed off. This degeneration could cause many cognitive and behavioral changes in the individuals that partake in excess drinking rituals. The neurodegeneration induced by alcoholism, which is often seen in chronic alcoholics, can be reduced through the use of CDB hemp oil.

Another study conducted by Mount Sinai School of Medicine also states that stimulus cue-induced in heroin addicts is lowered through the use of CBD hemp oil. The lowered stimuli can help to recover heroin addicts find an easier path to recovery with lesser relapses and cravings.

Moreover, CBD hemp oil can also reduce the symptoms of smoking marijuana, which has THC cannabinoid in excess. The Case study conducted by Department of Neuroscience and Behavior in University of São Paulo and INCT Translational Medicine showed that there was a decrease in the symptoms of the individual that was previously feeling marijuana withdrawals. It was concluded that CBD hemp oil could treat the complications such as loss of appetite, migraine, insomnia, anxiety, irritability, and other psychological issues in marijuana users.

Finally, another systematic review conducted on the intervention properties of CBD cannabinoid conducted by Université de Montréal concluded that CBD hemp oil could treat individuals with cocaine, opioid, and psychostimulant addiction. It was a clinical placebo study on individuals that were addicted to smoking and marijuana. Through some clinical studies and research done on the effects of CBD oil, it could be safely said that it can treat individuals struggling with various forms of addictive behaviors.

USE OF CBD HEMP OIL FOR ANXIETY DISORDERS

Mental health for each person is different; they have a different set of regular patterns of existence. The difference in the brain activity is the reason why anxiety disorders have so many medication dosages; it is also the reason why the dosage of this pharmaceutical medication is different for different people.

As above mentioned CBD hemp oil can help with various mental health disorders. It could help individuals quit smoking and other addictive habits as well. There is a different type of CBD hemp oil products available that could have the healing properties that have been mentioned above.

 The cannabinoids present in the CBD hemp oil have various properties that could be beneficial for the endocannabinoid system of the body. As it gives the endocannabinoid system of the body a boost and does not directly affect other systems of the body it does not have many side effects if taken in excess. There could be nausea or diarrhea, CBD hemp oil is taken in a very large quantity, which is very uncommon.

The cannabinoids travel on a molecular level through the pathways made by the receptors of the body. The receptors can move quickly through the blood, and the CBD can get carried to various parts of the body. It is easier for the body to take in the CBD hemp oil that is in contact with the bloodstream.

CBD oil is available in vapor form where it can be absorbed into the bloodstream from the lungs. This could give instant relaxation effects to the individuals that have had a panic attack or have gone through a stressful situation. This type of product does not give lasting effects; rather, it only gives momentary relief for one to two hours. The CBD oil may have some other lasting effects on the body such as its neuroprotective abilities and so forth. However, for long-lasting effects of CBD hemp oil, it is often recommended to take other strains of hemp oil in tincture or concentrated form. Some strains like Charlotte's web have been popular as a quick-acting medicine for anxiety attacks and epileptic issues.

The tincture form of CBD hemp oil can be taken as a regular supplement; it should hold under the tongue for a few minutes then swallowed for quicker and long effects. Other forms of CBD hemp oil can be added into the daily regiments of individuals that struggle with anxiety disorders as a pill or an edible supplement.

More importantly, it should be noted that individuals that want to add CBD hemp oil as a daily supplement should start at a lower dosage and see the effects of the medicine themselves as it considered the best strategy. The best process of finding the right dosage to get the optimal effects of CBD is through trial and error that is why one should find their dosage with their age, weight, and health in mind.

CBD HEMP OIL AS AN ANTIPSYCHOTIC

Psychotic disorders are the most severe mental disorders that are localized under the umbrella term known as psychosis. These disorders cause extreme stress in the individuals that have diagnosed with it; it is also known to cause sensory experiences where the patient believes to hear and see things that are not there. Individuals with this disorder may get psychotic episodes during stressful situations. This experience is incredibly frightening and could the patient to lash out, hurting themselves and others in the process.

The most common disorder associated with psychosis is schizophrenia, which has a large spectrum of disorders and symptoms associated with it. The most common sign and symptoms that are seen in patients with schizophrenia are a hallucination, where they see or hear things that do not exist. These patients may get delusional, which would cause them to have a suspicion of things that catch their eye, they may also make false belief of unreal things. The patients with psychosis are often seen to have disorganized thought patterns and speech behavior, which may cause them to jump from topic to topic with no relation in between.

In some severe cases, they may also become catatonic and have difficulty in concentrating on their surroundings. The initial stages of this disorder may progress slowly and transition into something severe over time. In milder cases of psychosis, individuals may feel suspicions, develop anxiety issues, may have fault perceptions, become obsessive, have sleeping issues, and become depressed.

The hallucinatory episodes in a psychotic patient may affect the sense of taste, touch, smell, sound, or sight, most commonly patient hears sever voices talking or giving a commentary on their daily life. The cause of psychosis is not properly understood; there can be many other issues that could instigate the growth of the symptoms. It could be caused by changes in the brain as patients with psychosis have reduced grey matter.

This disorder may also be caused by hormone or sleeping issues as the composition of the brain may change during the situations. Other causes might be a bipolar disorder or genetic causes. The traditional treatment for psychotic disorders does not treat the issues completely; it may reduce the symptoms and cause other complications as it is chemically changing the composition of the brain. The treatment for this disorder has two stages, where the heavy dosage of medication is given to the patient for the psychotic episodes. The other stage offers long-term therapy with fast-acting medicines for relaxation and maintenance of the mental health.

Several experiments done on the effects of cannabis and the endocannabinoid systems has concluded that it has some properties that can reduce the symptoms associated with psychotic issues. Which is why Cannabis has been used for the treatment of mental health disorder for quite some time. It was used to treat mental health disorders in ancient times as well.

However, this treatment had been associated with other psychotic side effects that may cause other complications because the cannabinoid THC had psychostimulant effects on the users. If THC cannabinoid that caused this complication was taken out of Cannabis oil, then a better version of the herbal medical could be found.

The study of its constituents led us to the discovery of CBD oil that had some healing properties, including being an antipsychotic and anxiolytic drug. A study conducted by researchers in Brazil also concluded that CBD OIL could be used as a safe alternative treatment for schizophrenia and bipolar disorders. Through this study, they used animal models to determine the neurochemical and behavioral effects of CBD and the pharmacological medicine used for the treatment of psychosis. It was not that the CBD had almost the same anti-psychotic properties as the medicine with many other beneficial effects.

SCHIZOPHRENIA

Schizophrenia is a chronic mental health disorder that has many severe complications. It causes the individual diagnosed with this condition to lose their touch with reality. This disorder may also cause symptoms of other mental health disorders to originate. Individuals of the age sixteen to thirty are susceptible to develop schizophrenic properties; they may develop three categories of symptoms. The first set of symptoms do not have a severe effect on the biology of the body.

Patients with the schizophrenic disorder may have hallucinations that would cause them to see and hear things that are not there. They may get delusional and have disordered thought patterns. Other symptoms such as disorderly movement may occur in a patient with schizophrenia. The symptoms that may cause the individual to have severe effects on the body include having the flat affect, where the facial expression and the voice tone of the individual is void of any emotions or quirks. They may also feel difficulty in sustaining everyday activities and daily chores, which may cause them to have irregular sleeping and eating habits causing malnutrition.

This disorder also causes other cognitive symptoms in the patient such as difficulty understanding basic information in their surrounding as well as difficulty making decisions. They may also develop issues with their memory and have a hard time recognizing their surroundings. The treatment for this disease is the antipsychotic medicine that is given to the patient in liquid or pill form. This medicine may be taken daily or weekly for the effects to become permanent. However, most of these medications target the symptoms that have acutely affected the individual's ability to live. They are given additional psychological treatment that includes therapy and counseling for them to have normal lifestyle and habits.

Other factors such as eating habits and sleeping irregularities are taken care of more medication or therapy. However, all of these issues could be treated through the proper use of CBD hemp oil after the client has been diagnosed. CBD cannabinoid present in the oil is a fast-acting antipsychotic, it could instantly provide relaxation if taken properly. CBD increases the production of anandamide receptors in the endocannabinoid system of the body. The increased levels of this receptor in the cerebrospinal fluid can reduce the symptoms associated with psychosis.

A research study conducted by Department of Psychiatry and Psychotherapy in Heidelberg University by several researchers also credited the antipsychotic effects of CBD hemp oil. This study was conducted by giving half the participant patients diagnosed with schizophrenia regular dosage of CBD oil, while the other was given a potent antipsychotic pharmaceutical medication known as amisulpride.

Both of the medication alleviated the symptoms associated with the mental health disorder. However, there was a difference in the side-effect profile of the two medications. The pharmaceutical medication showed many other adverse side effects in the mental health of the individuals, whereas, CBD oil had considerably lower side effects than it. This CBD oil also had better increase in the anandamide levels in the cerebral area, which led to the improvement of many other mental health issues. This research concluded that the increased levels of the anandamide in the brain could have antipsychotic effects on the mental health, which could be achieved through the use of CBD oil.

BIPOLAR PSYCHOSIS

Individuals diagnosed with Bipolar Psychosis have extreme mood swings that are attributed with bipolar disorders. During these extreme mood swings, psychotic episodes can occur that can cause the patient to have a delusional or disconnected view of the reality. These mood swings could cause the individual to become a danger to themselves and to those that surround them, as it can lead the patient to become angry with no reason and even have hallucinatory episodes about the people that care and support them. This type of mental health disorder is also known as manic depression. T

he main symptoms associated with the episodes during stressful situations are almost the same as schizophrenia, where the individual hallucinates and grandeur delusion of unreal things. The individual suffering from this disorder may also have confused thought patterns and extreme behavior.

Other symptoms of this mood disorder include episodes of depression that are followed by episodes of extreme highs known hypomanic episodes. During these episodes, the individuals may feel euphoric feelings that would be followed by extremely depressive state, which could cause the individual to have suicidal thoughts. Some individuals are misdiagnosed with schizophrenia when they have bipolar psychosis. The episodes of bipolar psychosis last a very small amount of time and are followed by manic episodes. Whereas, the episodes in schizophrenia last for a very long time.

CBD hemp oil could also have other nutritional benefits for individuals that suffer from mental health disorders. Often this disorder would have associated conditions such as irregularity in the daily diet as well as the sleeping regiment. CBD hemp oil has the necessary components to help with those issues as well. The hemp oil has many healthy fatty acids that could help with keeping the body in a healthy state, which might help individuals stay in a better mental state. The CBD cannabinoid connects with the CB1 receptors in the body to boost the endocannabinoid system that maintains the balance of many systems of the body.

By keeping a balance of the endocannabinoid system, the overall, anxiety and stress on the body could be reduced. Mental stress could cause individuals to have an irregular sleeping pattern as well, which can irritate mental health of a patient with acute conditions such as schizophrenia or bipolar psychosis.

CBD hemp oil has CBN cannabinoid that can improve the sleeping habits of the individuals as it has anti-insomniac properties. All in all, the properties such as antipsychotic, anti-insomnia, and anxiolytic that are readily available in CBD hemp oil can help patients that suffer from complicated mental health disorders.

SUBSTANCE-INDUCED PSYCHOSIS

Psychosis caused as a result of some medication or substance abuse is diagnosed as Substance-Induced Psychosis. This type of psychosis could cause individuals to have two types of major symptoms such as hallucination and delusions. Sometimes, individuals with this disorder may feel both of the disorders and other times; they would feel only one of the symptoms. These major symptoms are mostly diagnosed together as a substance-induced psychosis in substance abusers and individuals that take psychotic medication.

Other symptoms that may or may not appear are abnormal social behavior and a varied range of other psychological issues that may cause irregular emotions. Intoxication could cause the individuals to have a psychotic episode; it could also be caused by withdrawal. This psychotic breakdown is the reason individuals go through a detoxification process in severe cases of addiction or dependency disorders.

This psychosis could be caused by some substances such as cannabis, alcohol, inhalant, hallucinogens, sedatives, anxiolytics, hypnotics, amphetamines, cocaine, and other similar chemical drugs. The medication that could cause a psychotic attack on individuals could be an anesthetic, anticholinergic, antihistamine, anticonvulsant, cardiovascular, antiparkinsonian, chemotherapeutic, corticosteroid, gastrointestinal, muscle relaxant, and anti-inflammatory medication.

The abuse of this medication and drugs could cause pre-psychosis symptoms such as irritability, decreased attention span, sensitivity to light, sound, and touch, seizures, sudden mood changes, confusion/disorientation, delirium, body tremors, changes in mental functions, fatigue or stupor, and restlessness. Long-term substance abuse and dependency disorders in individuals could also cause the addicts to have psychotic breakdowns. Previously, CBD help oil had been suggested as a treatment for addiction and dependency disorders; it also can provide relief to smokers through various properties.

CBD hemp oil has the properties that could counteract the psychosis caused by other psychostimulants. There are many other cannabinoids in the CBD oil constituent that provide stress relieving and neuroprotective abilities. It relaxes the individual while inhibiting the properties of any other psychostimulants acting in the body. Moreover, CBD hemp oil has also been used as a treatment for substance abuse because of its neuroprotective abilities.

The active abilities of CBD cannabinoid have also given the medical world a path to renew treatment for psychotic disorders that had no previous symptoms. Under these circumstances, CBD hemp oil would be quite beneficial for individuals that have received treatment for the substance-induced psychotic disorder. By adding CBD oil as a supplement in the diet, these individuals can achieve a stable state of mind that can lead to a healthier body.

USE OF CBD HEMP OIL AS AN ANTIPSYCHOTIC

Each person has a different constitution and should decide their dosage with a few things in mind such as the weight, age, and their health. CBD hemp oil does not have many side effects, the cannabinoids present in this type of oil do not have psychoactive abilities. It is not supposed to make the individual that consumed it high, which is why it is impossible to overdose on this product. Unlike the pharmaceutical mental health medicine, CBD oil could be completely harmless if given to the patients with mental illness as it cannot be consumed to harm themselves during an episode.

There is some type of CBD that could be used to reduce the anxiety and stress during an episode and give long-lasting psychological effects on the body. One of the most common forms of CBD hemp oil is found in the form of tinctures. This type of product has the most concentrated form and can be found as pure CBD oil. Most manufacturers do not add any additives in tinctures so that it has maximum properties without being deluded by others. At times, some flavoring is added to the tincture to make the process of consuming it a little easier.

The dosage of tincture for people that need relief from the anxiety and stress from their lives could range from 100mg to 900 mg; it depends upon the concentration and the individual health. It is important to take small dosages of the product and move up higher if needed. Tinctures are usually held under the tongue or dropped on the tongue, where they are supposed to rest for a while before consuming. The resting allows the tincture to be absorbed into the bloodstream through the tongue.

The strongest dose of CBD hemp oil that could be obtained is in the form of CBD concentrate, which at times is ten times as stronger as other CBD hemp oil products. The CBD concentrate in comparison to tinctures is far easier to handle as they only take a few seconds to consume. The concentrated form of CBD hemp oil could be used in severe case of psychosis to help the patient relax after an episode. This type of oil does not have any type of additives; it may also lack the nutritional content of the hemp oil as it is the concentrate of CBD. It can consume the same way as a CBD tincture, by placing under a tongue and holding it a few minutes before consuming it.

The easiest way to consume CBD hemp oil is through capsules; it can be added as a supplement to the daily lives of the individual. The dosage of pills is already decided. Usually, they are offered in 10 to 25 mg of CBD hemp oil. This amount helps the individuals to slowly add this pill into the routine without causing a shock to the system. The daily serving allows individuals to add the CBD hemp capsule to their daily regiment with ease to provide many nutritional benefits.

It is also available as a topical treatment. However, this would only work to reduce the pain and skin issues of the individuals. If the mental health patient suffers from headaches and migraines, it could be used to apply in the affected area to help reduce the amount of pain. CBD has the ability of micellization that allows it to move through the skin layers into the body to provide its benefits. CBD oil infused products do not have as many effects as other products; they should be taken to reduce mild issues such as body ache, headache, or skin issues.

Another easier alternative to concentrates and tinctures is to use CBD hemp oil spray, this type of product does not have much concentration of CBD. It could be used throughout the day in any situations due to its availability. The amount of concentrate available in this sort of product range from 1 to 3 mg. This type of product could be beneficial for individuals with social anxiety and general anxiety disorder. As the spray can be used numerous times in the day to get minor anxiolytic effects to deal with the mild mental health issues such as anxiety and stress.

The quickest form of application or intake of CBD hemp oil is through vaporization. The amount of CBD taken through this process varies as the administration depends upon the amount of time the individual smokes. This type of product could be beneficial for addicts as it can give a little leeway to their smoking habits providing better alternatives. This type of product could be consumed numerous times a day. However, the absorption of the product may vary from person to person. CBD hemp oil is available for vaporization in vape pen, e-cigarettes, and inhalers.

Other edible products are also available that can give a minor helping hand to the individual suffering from mental health issues. CBD hemp oil is available as gums or candies so they can be easily ingested, it is also available as a patch for quicker application. It is important for individuals to find out a CBD hemp oil product that suits their needs, it should be noted that individuals with varied weight would have different recommended dosage.

A person that has mild mental health disorder with the weight of thirty to sixty lbs. Should take 2 to 4 mg plus of CBD oil. A person with 61 to 100 pounds. Weight should ingest 4 to 6 mg plus of the oil. A person with the weight of 100 to 175 lbs. Should swallow 6mg to 8mg of oil and a person of weight 175 to 250 lbs. should ingest 8 to 10mg of the oil. On the other spectrum, a person that suffers from severe mental health disorders with the weight of 31 to 60 lbs. should take 12 to 18 mg plus of CBD oil. A person with 61 to 100 lbs. weight should ingest 18 to 24 mg plus of the oil. A person with the weight of 100 to 175 lbs. should ingest 24mg to 32mg of oil and a person of weight 175 to 250 lbs. should ingest 32 to 40mg of the oil.

CHAPTER FIVE - CBD STRAINS AND EXTRACTS

Before diving in the different types of CBD strains and extracts, let review the differences between CBD cannabinoid and THC cannabinoid. The CBD cannabinoid does not have any psychostimulant abilities; it does not have the symptoms of mild altering high. CBD could be taken from the plants in various concentrations with other mixture of cannabinoids. Sometimes, it is mixed with THC with the ratio being in CBD's favor. This type of CBD hemp oil does not contain any high effects that would be associated with THC as the concentration would be really low.

CBD cannabinoid can connect with the receptors in the endocannabinoid system of the body to provide various effects to deal with emotions, mood, pain, movement, and other disorders. On the other hand, like other cannabinoids THC or delta9-tetrahydrocannabinol can also connect with the endocannabinoid receptors and produce psychoactive effects in the brain. The effects of THC are usually short-term as it can cause instant euphoria and reduced anxiety in the individual. It may also give the user increased appetite for a limited time.

Various strains are made from High CBD cannabis extracts, which has the best of properties of both THC and CBD. In these strains, the amount of THC is very low, which is why these strains have now boomed in the medical community. Some of the strains that are popular in the community are Cannatonic, Harlequin, Harle-Tsu, ACDC, CBD Critical Cure, Charlotte's Web, Canna-Tsu, One to One, and Sour Tsunami. The ratio of the strains mentioned above varies to give different effects on the body. Moreover, these strains are taken from the high CBD extract, where other types of extracts that have no THC content also exist.

TYPES OF EXTRACT

There are many different types of extracts that use different hemp plants to get various effects. The CBD products have some Cannabinoid constituents that could vary in these extracts. Depending upon the type, it might be a full spectrum CBD extract or a High dosage CBD extract. Each of these extracts has a different chemical makeup that designs specific products aimed at various issues.

HIGH-CBD OIL

The high CBD oil has only one difference from the CBD hemp oil, which is recommended in most cases, which is the THC ratio, or none to be exact. Both of these extracts are taken from the same species of the Sativa plant; they are both given the same treatment.

However, the high CBD hemp oil would have a concentration of 0.3 THC or lower, which is the legal amount of THC that is medically approved. The strains made from this type oil need a medical certificate for access as most federal laws considers it illegal for daily use. The stains that could be made from this oil are Cannatonic, Harlequin, Harle-Tsu, ACDC, CBD Critical Cure, Charlotte's Web, Canna-Tsu, One to One, and Sour Tsunami.

CBD HEMP OIL

This type of CBD oil is very common in the industry and has been used to produce various products for easier dosage. This oil is made by pressing the seeds and stems of the hemp plant to get the various beneficial properties. However, the creation of this type of oil is very easy and makes the production of low-grade CBD oil products an imminent factor.

Some industries use the proper medical and naturally grown plants to provide concentrated dosages of CBD hemp oil. This oil could be used to make strains. However, the effects may vary. The THC contents of this oil are very low and close to none, which is why it is suited as a better alternative for long-term issues and disorders that affects the daily lives of the individuals. This type of CBD is available in different type of products that offer suitability and taste for the liking of the consumer. The CBD hemp oil products range from tinctures, concentrates, capsules, topical creams, balms, shampoos, skincare products, candies, and other edible products.

TYPES OF STRAINS

Some strains that have a low THC content and a high CBD content can help individuals that suffer from acute to severe disorders. One of the most popular strains that work best for children is Charlotte's Web, which has a mixed ratio of THC and CBD. It could treat severe epileptic conditions and depressive disorders.

Moreover, the high dosages of CBD in these strains cancels out the effects of THC, making them one of the best treatments for acute social anxiety disorders, depressive disorders, panic disorders, general anxiety disorders, epileptic disorders, and other similar conditions. Let us take a close look at the different strains and effects.

CHARLOTTE'S WEB

Charlotte's Web is one of the most popular and well-known strains in the medical world. This strain is taken from the Sativa hybrid plant that has no psychoactive constituents. The focus of this strain was to create a legalized CBD oil strain to help individuals with acute epileptic seizures. The ratio of the THC cannabinoid and CBD cannabinoid in this strain is the reason that this strain is very popular among people. The ratio of CBD and THC in this strain is 20:1, where the THC cannabinoid has an extremely low concentration of THC. This allows this strain to be sold in other CBD products as well. Individuals that consume this strain do not feel any pain associated with the typical psychoactive cerebral effect.

This strain is known to offer relief to epileptic disorders such as Dravet's syndrome. This strain has powerful constituents that give it anxiolytic abilities. It also offers relief for other issues such as a headache, fatigue, epilepsy, depression, anxiety, pain, seizures, stress, and muscle spasms. This strain is also being used to bring creative, uplifting, relaxed, happy, and focused feelings in mental health patients that have mild to moderate depressions and anxiety issues.

The history behind this strain goes along like this, in 2013, a girl named Charlotte Figi was suffering from Dravet syndrome. The pharmaceutical drugs prescribed to her had little to no effect, which is why their parents sought out cannabis extract to help their daughter. After using this extract, the frequency of charlottes epileptic seizures dropped from approximately 100 a week to a few times a month. This astonishing discovery led to the further study of this strain and many other strains that could potentially become an herbal remedy for untreatable disorders.

ACDC

This hybrid strain has one the largest percentage ratio of CBD to THC, where there is the CBD content might be 20% and the THC content 6%. This THC percentage can be as low as 0.42%, which is greater than the legal percentage of THC. This is the reason that ACDC cannot be found in CBD oil form, it is not accessible to the masses. Some states allow access to this strain after obtaining a medical card that is given after a complete checkup of the medical background of the individual.

Being a high CBD strain, it has potent properties that could help with stress, seizures, pain, nausea, inflammation, epilepsy, cancer, anxiety, Parkinson's, multiple sclerosis, muscle spasms, cramps, and arthritis. This type of strain is known to bring a euphoric, relaxed, uplifting, happy, and focused mood changes without any psychoactive effects in the individual ingesting it. This type of strain is derived from the Sativa plant that has a parent lineage with the cannatonic marijuana strain.

This strain has many active and quick acting properties that could give instant relief to epileptic patients as well as individuals suffering from acute psychosis. This strain is also known to mitigate the aftereffects of chemotherapy in cancer patients.

CANNA-TSU

Canna-Tsu is a mix between to other high CBD strains known as a cannatonic and sour tsunami. Both of the parent strains are known to offer an upbeat feeling after use; it does not have psychoactive high. Canna-Tsu has the same amount of CBD and THC ratio; it generally offers pain relief and mood elevation properties after ingestion.

At times, the amount of CBD is higher than the THC to counteract against any of the psychoactive effects of the later constituent of cannabis. This type of strain has a woody taste and aroma. However, it may be accentuated with spicy or citrus flavors to be made pleasing to tongue and nose of the user.

It gives the users a focused, euphoric, relaxed. Social, uplifting, and an energetic mood that often brings a laid-back experience to the user. It could also offer relief for various disorders such as anxiety, migraines, muscle spasms, nausea, stress, spasticity, inflammation, Parkinson's, pain, muscular dystrophy, multiple sclerosis, gastrointestinal disorder, depression, and ADD/ADHD among others.

Canna-Tsu is also known as the happy-go-lucky strain as it brings an uplifting feeling as well as mild analgesic effects. This type of strain would be beneficial for individuals suffering from depressive mood disorders as it can keep the user in a happy and easy-going mood for some time. The scent, as mentioned above, has refreshing quality because of its parent hybrids that have a sweet and woody scent. Associated with the scent is the taste that is associated with sour pine and sweet citrus, it also has a mix of earthy and woody aftertaste. This strain may cause the user to have a parched mouth and dryness eyes.

SOUR TSUNAMI

This strain of high-CBD has the same ratio of CBD and THC cannabinoid in the constituents. Their ratio is nearly considered 1:1 in the medical community. This strain was introduced in Humboldt by a company named Southern Humboldt Seed Collective. The person that bred this strain was aiming to develop an herb that could lower the pain felt by opioid addiction recovery, which led it is a great alternative to pain medication given to patients with opioid addiction.

Some markets sell Sour Tsunami strain that has more CBD content than the THC content. No matter which consistency, this strain is considered to have a strong pain relieving property. It is consumed recreationally and by patients suffering from various disorders because of this pain relieving and mood enhancing abilities.

Sour Tsunami is a friendly strain that can be used dry for beginners to have a relaxed and calm introduction to CBD strains. This strain has more THC than the legalized limit, which is why it cannot be bought without a medical card. This strain can be found as a flower, as a tincture, or in an oil form to suit the needs of the individual. This strain has an earthy aroma that has notes of citrus and harp pine because of the existence of limonene and pinene.

This strain has also been associated with the entourage effect, which offers modulating abilities to many parts of the body so it can recover proper balance and health. This strain is known to cause a focused, sleepy, uplifting, happy, and relaxed feeling without the euphoric high that could hinder the daily lives of the individuals. The psychoactive abilities of the sour tsunami have been claimed to be very mild and close to non-existent. Individuals with multiple sclerosis and seizure disorders have found this train to have optimum pain relieving and stress reducing abilities.

The Sour Tsunami strain is also popular in individuals that have inflammatory disorders such as arthritis and fibromyalgia. Due to the high levels of CBD and very low amount of THC, this strain can also mitigate the complications associated with anxiety disorders. Moreover, this strain can also inhibit the cannabis-induced anxiety that is common in marijuana users. All in all, it can provide relief to the patients suffering from stress, anxiety, pain, muscle spasms, multiple sclerosis, migraines, insomnia, headaches, epilepsy, cramps, arthritis, and fibromyalgia.

CANNATONIC

Cannatonic is a High-CBD strain that was made by the Spanish seed bank Resin Seeds because of it lower THC ratio. The ratio of THC and CBD cannabinoid in the cannatonic strain is 1:3, respectively. The percentage of the THC content could be as high as 6%, whereas, the percentage of the CBD content could be as high as 17%. It is known to produce a mellow and relaxing feeling in the individual. The relaxing feeling is felt both in mind and the body of the individual consuming it, which is why it is a great alternative for individuals that have chronic pain and epilepsy disorders. This strain can be found in various forms like a tincture, oil, or as a flower, which could be smoked to have the relaxing effects.

 The relaxing power of cannatonic has a potent ability to bring numbing and warm sensations in the body that can work effectively for individuals that suffer from migraines, headaches, and mood disorders. The high associated with this strain is not long lasting as the THC content is very low, whereas, the other relaxing and pain relieving effects of this strain are long lasting and can provide relief throughout the body. The Sativa strain is more dominant in this strain that is why it can affect the cognitive and mood of the individual. This strain has an herbal aroma that has a touch of citrus and woody scent. It has a light green color with darker pistils that attribute a dense and airy experience during smoking.

This strain can combat the pain that is felt by migraines and headaches. Other disorders such as Parkinson's. Multiple sclerosis and epilepsy may be treated by this strain. Some individuals have claimed that this strain leaves them with a dry mouth and feelings of paranoia. All in all the cannatonic strain could help individuals with Tourette's syndrome, stress, spinal cord injury, spasticity, seizures, PTSD, PMS, phantom limb pain, Parkinson's, pain, nausea, muscular dystrophy, muscle spasms, multiple sclerosis, migraines, inflammation, headaches, glaucoma, gastrointestinal disorder, fibromyalgia, eye pressure, epilepsy, depression, Crohn's disease, cramps, arthritis, bipolar disorder, Alzheimer's and anxiety.

HARLEQUIN

Harlequin is another popular CBD high strain that has a unique CBD: THC ratio. The ratio of this strain can be simply described to 5:2, where the CBD levels can be as high as 6 % and the THC levels could be as high as 16 percent. This strain is associated with relaxing and calming feeling that leaves the individual alert and focused as an aftereffect. By the other strains found, Harlequin is considered a mildly effective strain.

Harlequin strain has uplifting mood abilities that could provide energetic, happy, relaxed, focused, pain relieving, and uplifting feeling in the consumer. This strain provides the pain relieving and relaxing feeling to the consumer without the associated psychoactive high. The greater amount of CBD allows the individual consuming this strain have ample amounts of clarity with a relaxing feeling. It has potent mood-lifting abilities that could be beneficial or individuals that suffer from mood disorders.

This strain is considered a good starting point for individuals that have not used other cannabis strains. The popularity of High CBD strain in the market is varied due to the aroma, scent, and the flavors of different strains as well as the potency of the strains.

Harlequin strain has been associated with the mango flavor due to the fruitiness lurking underneath the visage. Other scents like woody and citric scent also contribute to its aroma. The smoke of this strain is smooth and does not linger on the tongue. The color of this strain is mid-greenish with a thick layer of orange pistils that may have a sticky look. Harlequin has been popular in the market due to its versatility; it is used both by recreational users as well as medical consumers. The properties of this strain can help with the neuropathic pain associated with multiple sclerosis and Parkinson's. It can provide a happy and uplifting feeling that is why individuals suffering from mild anxiety disorders as well PTSD may find it beneficial for their condition.

This strain is used to produce oils and extracts that are targeted to give relief and relaxation in the body that could be beneficial for acute muscle spasms and seizure disorders. All in all, the harlequin strain could be beneficial for individuals that from stress, seizures, PTSD, phantom limb pain, Parkinson's, pain, muscle spasms, multiple sclerosis, migraines, inflammation, headaches, fibromyalgia, fatigue, epilepsy, depression, bipolar disorders, arthritis, and anxiety.

HARLE-TSU

Harle-Tsu is comparable to ACDC due to its CBD: THC ratio, this strain features twenty times more CBD content than that of THC. The THC percentage in this strain is very low that is why it is often considered a might High CBD strain. However, the percentage of the THC in this strain is still higher than that of the legal limit (0.3%). This strain is available as medical cannabis at dispensaries, individuals with a medical car can easily access this strain. This non-psychoactive strain is popular in individuals that suffer from acute anxiety and pain disorders.

This strain is a mix between Harlequin and Sour Tsunami that has resulted in the production of a strain that has 20 times more CBD cannabinoid then the THC cannabinoid. The lower levels of THC attribute this strain a very low and non-existent levels of psychoactive properties. This strain is known to have an earthy and woody aroma, where there are a sharp spicy and pine-like sent to the buds. Others have also attributed a citrus-like scent and a sweetened scent. This strain is found in the form of concentrates and oil; many individuals enjoy the use of this strain because of its medical and recreational properties. This strain has been attributed to having a relaxing feeling that can take the edge of the daily lives. It can also reduce the stress that is common among patients that have mental health disorders.

Individuals that have chronic pain issues are often seen to opt for this strain as it as potent analgesic abilities that could deal with chronic pain. This strain can also give individuals that had a restless night a more alert and focused feeling. Some individuals have also claimed that Harlequin has the abilities similar to that of aspirin as both of them relieve pain without any high.

It does not cause the individuals to have a body-heavy sensation; rather, it promotes the loosening of stiff muscles and joints through its strong relaxation properties. This strain is known to produce focused, relaxed, uplifting, and happy feeling in the individuals. All in all, this strain could help individuals that suffer from mild anxiety disorders, mood disorders, stress, pain, chronic pain, headache, cramps, migraines, inflammation, PTSD, insomnia, arthritis, and depression.

RINGO'S GIFT

Ringo's Gift is a mixture of the two very popular strain's known as ACDC and Harle-Tsu, both of which have a high CBD percentage then THC. The ratio of the cannabinoids is very much like its parent strains, where the ratio of CBD: THC is 24:1. This contrast in the percentage allows it to have the benefits of both cannabinoids as well as near to none psychoactive properties. This strain offers a mellow and soothing relaxation to the consumer without the "couch lock" effect that causes euphoria and hunger.

The smell of this strain has a very fresh and delicate aroma that has undertones of mint. The taste of this strain corresponds to the smell of as it as has an earthy flavor with a minty tang when you exhale the smoke; the minty tang intensifies as you smoke it. The color of the strain is light green, and the buds have a light neon green color with orange fuzz. The mellow properties of this strain give soothing effects to the cerebral region and the body. The sensation of this strain leaves the individual feeling social and happy as it has potent powers that offer relief of physical and mental pain. This allows the individual consuming the strain to become focused and motivated enough to complete the task in a calm headspace.

This of strain works best for individuals that suffer from anxiety and stress-related disorders as it is known to produce a mellow feeling. Patients that have anxiety, depression, PTSD, insomnia, psychosis, and epilepsy may find this strain helpful as it offers a potent body relaxation effects that start from head to toe, slowly melting the worries away. Ringo's gift is popular among individuals that suffer from PTSD, stress, muscle spasms, gastrointestinal disorder, arthritis, anxiety, and chronic pain.

ONE TO ONE

One to One is one of the strains that often overlooked because of the CBD and THC levels in its constitution. The levels of CBD and THC are about the same that is why this strain may cause slightly subtle psychoactive effects on the consumer. This hybrid strain is bred by stabilizing the High CBD landrace strain and Amnesia Haze (a potent strain well known because of its mood-lifting abilities). This hybrid is known to give calming effects on individuals suffering severe mental health issues.

This strain can also increase the creativity and focus of the individuals using it. It brings an easygoing effect on the individual by brig relief from the stress and anxiety. This strain has potent properties of both CBD cannabinoid and THC cannabinoid, where the percentage of this cannabinoid can range up to 14%. Most CBD high strains are known to be medically used to provide relief to the individuals, one to one is no exception to this rule. This strain offers a mild pain relieving effect on the individual more than the high. The buzz received through this strain brings a blissful and happy uplifting feeling in the individual that does not cause them to become sedated or have the "couch-lock" effect.

One to One, like many other CBD high strains, has an earthy aroma with hints of woody and nutty scent. Being a potent strain of CBD, it has many therapeutic effects on the users. It is popularly used by individuals that need to reduce the amount of pain felt during chronic pin episodes and inflammatory disorders. It also has potent ant-epileptic properties, which is why it is often used by individuals that suffer from severe seizure and mental health issues. The high amount of CBD and THC content offers a relaxation effect in the body that relaxes the muscles and joints during spasm attacks in the patient suffering from Dravet's syndrome.

By rounding up all of the properties that offer beneficial effects, it is concluded that individuals suffering from stress, spinal cord injury, spasticity, seizures, PMS, phantom limb pain, Parkinson's, pain, muscular dystrophy, muscle spasms, multiple sclerosis, migraines, lack of appetite, inflammation, headaches, fibromyalgia, depression, bipolar disorders, arthritis, anxiety, and ADD can find relief by using One on One strain.

CBD CRITICAL CURE

CBD Critical Cure was made with the promise of bringing a medically beneficial strain that could provide rapid mood lifting and analgesic effects. This strain has been used as a mild sedative in the medical world; it does not have any psychoactive effects. It promises to give the consumer positive mood-lifting effects that rapidly provide a relaxing and calming effect on the mind and the body.

CBD Critical Cure was produced in the West Coast from a parent strain known as Critical Kush. The resulting strain provided a low THC bud that had sedative abilities that could be used to treat various disorders of the body. This strain, like the name suggests, offers a higher ration of CBD and a very low ratio of THC. The CBD levels of this strain can range from 8 to 12 % in approximately, whereas, the THC strain almost always has a 5% or lower THC levels.

 It does not have any psychoactive abilities because of the higher levels of CBD. However, some part of the THC still shows effects such as the sedative properties of this strain. This strain has a sweet and pine-like scent; there is a sharp contrast with a fruity scent that is a bit pungent. The taste of this strain has an earthy quality and a sweet aftertaste. This strain can be used as a mild herbal tranquilizer due to its sedation effects. It provides a pleasant and gentle relaxing feeling in the body that can uplift the spirits. Many individuals use this strain for recreational purposes; other use it for medical purposes.

Individuals that suffer from anxiety, depression, post-traumatic stress disorder, and other related issues could find relief and relaxation by using this strain. The mixture of the two cannabinoids in this strain allows it to become a powerful pain management system. It could be used by individuals with inflammatory conditions such as gastrointestinal disorders and arthritis. The mild sedation effects of this strain may also help individuals with insomnia find a manageable sleeping routine.

CALI CURE

Cali Cure is one of the CBD high strains that could provide an energetic and uplifting feeling to the individual with mild sedation effects. This strain has a higher concentration of CBD than THC. The CBD levels of this strain can range up to 15%, and the THC strain can range up to 7%, this keeps a 2:1 ratio of the two cannabinoids respectively. This strain is known to have a citric scent with undertones of pine-like aroma. The taste attributed to this strain develops from the smell, which provides a lemony and spicy aftertaste to the smoke.

This strain has also won the Best CBD Flower award in the Southern California Cannabis Cup in 2016. Cali Cure is particularly known to provide energizing effects to the user as well as a light dosage of sedation that lower the risk of anxiety attacks or other mental episodes. Other properties of this strain include providing an uplifting, social, relaxing, and creative feeling.

This type of strain has a higher dosage of THC level than some of the other strains, which is why it will have a slightly mild "couch lock" on the user. It advised using this herb after work hours to relax the mind and the body after strenuous hours. This strain is also a potent pain reliever and can help individuals that have inflammatory and chronic pain disorders. It is also is known to induce appetite so individuals that have eating disorders could also find appetite stimulant effects through this strain. Canna cure also has a [potent mood stabilizing ability that could provide a balanced mood to individuals that suffer from depression and anxiety disorders.

DESERT RUBY

Desert Ruby is another High CBD strain that has won Best CBD Concentrate awards and Best CBD Flower in the Denver Cannabis Cups. This strain demonstrates a top-shelf level of CBD ratio in its constituents. This strain is well known in the Colorado region as it was localized in that area. This strain has strong pain relieving and relaxing effects on the individual. It can help people that have anxiety disorders find a calmer headspace. Due to the higher concentration of CBD, it can help with many disorders.

Desert Ruby displays a potent buzz that brings relaxation to the body from head to toe; this relaxation allows the mind maintain a care-free attitude. This type of strain can be used by individuals that need to unwind and relax so they can sleep in peace. It is also used as a recreational herb because of its relaxation effects. Its constituents allow the behavior of the consumer to become motivated and uplifted. Having a high level of cannabinoid content makes this herb, not a perfect drug to consume in the daytime.

It is advised that individuals smoke this herb after their work hours as it is known to bring a relaxation effect to help individuals suffering stress and anxiety disorders. It also has a mild analgesic effect so patients that have chronic pain and inflammation disorders can find relief through the use of this strain. All in all, this strain can help relieve the symptoms of various issues such as anxiety, depression, PTSD, inflammation, pain, and epilepsy.

REMEDY

The remedy is one of those High CBD strains that have almost close to none THC levels, whereas, the CBD levels are as high as 15%. This allows both of the cannabinoids to become active constituents of the strains. The parent strains of Remedy are the hybrid strain cannatonic and the indicia strain known as Afghan skunk. Due to the lower levels of THC in this strain, there no psychoactive effect on the consumer.

The buds of this strain have a yellow color and have shiny exterior. This strain has a floral scent that allows the user to fall into a mellow state. This state works in a benefit for individuals that are looking for a relaxation effect in the body and the mind. Many consumers have claimed that this strain is the perfect alternative to pharmaceuticals that they use for their sleeping and anxiety disorders. This strain has a flower, woody, and earthy smell, along with a slight citrus taste.

It provides relaxation to the user as well as a happy and uplifting feeling that could stabilize any mood disorders. It is a potent sleep stimulant and can help individuals that have trouble sleeping. It also has potent pain relieving properties as well as relaxing effect on the body. It helps relieves the stress from the muscles and the joints so that the individual has a stress free time. This strain is known to cause a dry mouth in the consumers. Remedy strain would be beneficial for individuals that suffer from pain, seizures, autism, inflammation, anxiety disorders, and depression.

DANCEHALL

DanceHall has a unique proportion of THC and CBD content as the average ratio of these cannabinoids can be 1:20, respectively. This strain is a Sativa dominant hybrid that was bred from the parent strains known Kalijah and Juanita La Lagrimosa, both of which have Mexican-Afghani ancestry.

Dancehall can have a gradual effect on the consumer that brings a potent uplifting and creative feeling in the individual along with many beneficial effects. This strain could cause the individual to have an easier time at social gatherings. The flower of this plant has a vibrant purple, green, to a blue color with undertones red. The aroma and taste of this strain are associated with a sweet and spicy flavor. The flavor comes from earthy textures, with the pepper-like aftertaste.

Due to the high CBD and lower THC levels, it has the best properties of both strains without causing psychoactive effects. It causes the individual to feel happy and relaxed, through which they feel a creative and uplifting feeling. This potency of this strain also allows it to have strong analgesic and anxiolytic effects on the body. The individual that suffer from acute mental health and pain disorders could find instant and long-lasting relief to the body and the mind. It is also known to reduce inflammation and the pain caused by a headache and migraines.

The individuals that have consumed this herb have associated its effects to cause dry mouth, dry eyes, and slight paranoia. By rounding up all of the properties that offer beneficial effects, it is concluded that individuals suffering from stress, spinal cord injury, spasticity, seizures, PMS, phantom limb pain, Parkinson's, pain, muscular dystrophy, muscle spasms, multiple sclerosis, migraines, lack of appetite, inflammation, headaches, fibromyalgia, depression, bipolar disorders, arthritis, anxiety, and ADD can find relief by using Dancehall strain.

SUZY Q

Suzy Q has a low THC ratio and a very high CBD ration that causes the consumer to have no psychoactive effects after uses. This strain was tested to have around 18% CBD and less than 1 % THC levels, which makes it the perfect alternative to anxiety pharmaceuticals taken in the daytime. The smell of this strain is spicy and pine-like, whereas, the taste associated with this strain is pepper-like and herbal.

This strain is known to be a potent relaxant and can provide stress-free day to the individual that use it at daytime. This strain also causes the individual to have the "munchies" so it can be used as an appetite stimulant for individuals that have eating disorders. Its effects are also known to cause very mild sedation that could help individuals relax in high-stress situations. The high CBD levels in this strain allow it to have a powerful analgesic effect, it could be used to relieve the symptoms associated with inflammation.

It has mild effects on headache and fatigue; mostly, it is used as a relaxant to provide a calm headspace to people that suffer from anxiety disorders. Consumers of this strain have stated that the use of this herb could cause dry mouth, dry eyes, and headaches. This type of strain could be used by individuals that need a mild analgesic for their pain and stress issues. Rounding it better properties up, it could be said that this strain can help individuals that have chronic pain, arthritis, muscle spasms, anxiety, and nausea.

DANCE WORLD

Dance World is a high CBD strain that is bred by crossbreeding the Dancehall and its parent strain Juanita La Lagrimosa. Dancehall is known to cause happy and uplifting feeling in the individual. Dance World inherits many of the better traits of its parents to offer mood stabilization effect on the user. This strain is effective against depressive disorders as it can produce a happy and relaxed feeling in the individual, along with uplifted and creative boost in the mood.

The aroma of this herb has uplifting scent associated with lavender and citrus, while its taste is known to be herbal/spicy and citrusy. Dance world, in particular, can be used by the patient that has stress issues as it has potent stress relieving properties. This strain can have a mild analgesic effect. It can help individuals that have inflammation and headaches. Mostly, this strain is used by the medical world to treat the stress-induced disorders and depressive disorders. This strain, like many other strains, is known to cause a dry mouth in the user. In conclusion, Dance world is most effects in individuals that suffer from depression, anxiety, PTSD, social anxiety disorders, and other anxiety-related issues.

CBD SHARK

CBD Shark is a mildly effective strain that has high CBD levels. This strain can help individuals with various issues such as inflammation and pain without any psychoactive effects. The smell of this strain is often compared to berries and citrus with a mild undertone of skunk-like smell; this aroma gives it an earthy and citrusy taste when smoked. This strain is known to offer relaxation to the user and induce happy and tingly sensations all over the body. Some individuals may also feel hungry or sleepy if this strain is used in excess. It has powerful analgesic properties that could relieve the symptoms of pain disorders.

CBD Shark can also reduce inflammation and help treat inflammatory disorders in the long term. This strain can offer stress relief due to its relaxing and mood stabilizing abilities; it could also contribute to the lower frequency of anxiety attacks in patients that suffer from anxiety-induced disorders. It can also deal with mild headaches due to its pain relieving properties. Consumers of this strain have often claimed that they have dry eyes and dry mouth after using this strain. Individuals that suffer from arthritis, migraines, anxiety, depression, inflammation will find CBD shark useful because of its beneficial properties.

PENNYWISE

Pennywise is a potent strain that high CBD levels and THC levels. This plant I an excellent alternative to inflammation and pain that is associated with severe medical issues. The total cannabinoids present in this strain are very high, which contributes to some beneficial properties to this strain. The ratio of CBD and THC in this strain are equal and can contribute to 30% of the cannabinoid constitution of the strain. This is crafted to offer potent abilities of both the cannabinoid that could help individuals suffering from severe health disorders.

The parent strain of Pennywise is Harlequin and Jack the Ripper. The flower of this plan has a purple and green color, whereas, the buds have a milky exterior. On average, this strain produced 10 to 15% of CBD and THC constituents to give a 1:1 of the cannabinoids. The aroma of this strain tends to change according to the growth environment; it usually has a bubblegum-like aroma.

The attributes to a sweet and woody taste while smoking, some consumers have also claimed that it has a sharp spicy smell like black pepper. Due to the high THC levels of this strain, it does have psychoactive properties. Otherwise, this strain provides a soft and mellow experience to the user along with the relaxation of the mind and body. It is not recommended to be inhaled during the daytime in excess; only light dosages could have a strong analgesic and many other beneficial properties. The sedative effects also make the consumer slightly sleepy, the effects have been associated with that of a chamomile tea.

Pennywise has a large number of cannabinoid content that could offer relaxation without overpowering the mind. This strain is considered to have a great relaxation effect after a strenuous day. The combination of CBD and THC allow this strain to have many therapeutic effects that could treat severe issues such as epilepsy, multiple sclerosis, cancer pain and many other issues. The anti-inflammatory abilities of this strain allow it to have potent abilities that could relieve the symptoms of depression, arthritis, and diabetes. Through the regular use of this drug, individuals can find effective treatment through its pain-relieving, anti-inflammatory, and antioxidant properties.

CORAZÓN

Corazón in an obscure and rare strain that has been bred by crossbreeding ACDC and Charlotte's Web strain. The parent strain gives it the best qualities as a medicinal strain because it has the highest CBD content ratio to that of the THC. This is the reason that makes it one of the best strains that could be marketed as a medicinal CBD treatment. The testing on the Corazón strain revealed that it had almost 23 % CBD content in it, while the THC percentage was between 2 to 3 %.

The percentage of CBD allows it to have many properties that could be beneficial for individuals that have severe disorders. This strain is derived from

Sativa dominant plant, which gives it potent medicinal properties and close to none psychoactive properties. By smoking this strain, the individual will receive a quick acting herb that will offer relief to individuals of all kinds. It brings the individual to a calm and happy space as they feel a warm and numbing sensation in their body.

Consumers have stated that this strain is known to have a citrusy and woody aroma and taste while being smoked. The analgesic properties of this strain could also help cancer patient find relief; it could even develop the parent properties to induce cancer reducing properties in the body. The strong effects of this smoke could also bring a relaxing effect on the individuals that could help the patient suffering from epileptic disorders. Corazon, like its parent strain, has powerful constituents that give it anxiolytic abilities. It also offers relief for other issues such as a headache, depression, anxiety, pain, seizures, fatigue, epilepsy, stress, and muscle spasms.

This strain is also being used to bring relaxed, happy, creative, uplifting, and focused feelings in mental health patients that have mild to severe anxiety disorders and other mental health issues. Being the most CBD High strain, it has potent properties that could help with severe stress, seizures, pain, nausea, Parkinson's, multiple sclerosis, inflammation, epilepsy, cancer, anxiety, muscle spasms, cramps, and arthritis.

VALENTINE X

Valentine X is one of the stronger strains, whose properties have been labeled on par with that of ACDC because of its potent and active constituents. This strain was made in California by balancing Sativa and Indica strains. Mainly, it was bred to have potent medicinal properties by selecting phenotypes of ACDC to enhance the beneficial properties further. The CBD profile of this strain found that it had gotten the parent strains of its ancestors such as OG Kush, G13, MK Ultra, Haze, G13 haze, Cannatonic, and ACDC.

The name of this strain stems from the St. Valentine, who was known to be the saint of love and marriage. However, St. Valentine was also the saint of epilepsy, he is more commonly associated with epilepsy in children and adolescents. This strain produces a smooth and mellow feeling in the consumer that is followed by a calming sensation of the body. Users of this strain have also stated that it brought a euphoric, happy, and relaxing feeling along with increased sociability and creativity.

The taste of this strain is associated with an earthy flavor that is amplified because of the presence of pinene, myrcene, and caryophyllene terpenes present in its constituents. It has a unique aroma that has hints of lemongrass and eucalyptus, bring the consumer an invigorating and energizing feeling. Being a potent source of many cannabinoids that could help individuals with various diseases, it can help treat pain, spasms, and sleep disorders.

This strain is also known to have antibacterial, anti-tumor, antiseptic properties due to the caryophyllene, which could help individuals suffering from cancer. This powerful strain could help individuals with Tourette's syndrome, seizures, PTSD, PMS, phantom limb pain, Parkinson's, pain, nausea, muscular dystrophy, migraines, inflammation, gastrointestinal disorder, headaches, glaucoma, fibromyalgia, eye pressure, epilepsy, depression, Crohn's disease, cramps, arthritis,stress, spinal cord injury, spasticity bipolar disorder, muscle spasms, multiple sclerosis, Alzheimer's and anxiety.

SPECIFIED STRAINS FOR VARIOUS DISORDERS

The number of strains that could be produced with Sativa and Indica plants can range over hundreds. It could be hard for individuals that need a specific strain for their issues. Some strains can be picked out to get in the right mindset and for its medical properties. Most of the strains to could affect the daily life of the individual by promoting moods and by providing medicinal properties are set as follows:

- *To uplift the spirit,* strains such as Cherry Pie, Mango Kush, Lemon Skunk, Bubbleberry, Pineapple Kush, Blue Magoo ,Snoop's Dream, Blue Haze, Blue Dragon, Pineapple Trainwreck, Lodi Dodi, Raskal OG, Blue Moon Rocks, Super Green Crack, Grape Kush, Blue Mystic, Timewreck, LA Chocolat, Secret Recipe, Hemlock, Pearl Scout Cookies, Jamaican, NYPD, Rollex OG Kush, Green Hornet, Viper,

Pineapple Super Silver Haze, The Sauce, GRiZ Kush, King Kong, Green Candy, Lucky Charms, FPOG, Purple Monkey Balls, Neville's Haze, Silver Kush, White Lightning, Jah Kush, Space Bomb, OG Cheese, Hawaiian Punch, White Urkle, Rockstar Kush, Critical Haze, White Lavender, Fire Alien Kush, Bubblicious ,Oregon Pineapple, Armageddonand, Super Sweet could be used.

- *To become energized*, strains such as Sour Diesel, Green Crack, Jack Herer, Pineapple Express, Durban Poison, AK-47, Lemon Haze, Strawberry Cough, Super Silver Haze, Alaskan Thunder Fuck, Super Lemon Haze, Amnesia Haze, Maui Wowie, Chocolope, Golden Goat, Agent Orange, Harlequin, Cinex, Cinderella 99, NYC Diesel, Candyland Cotton, Candy Kush, Tangerine Dream, Tangie, Lamb's Bread, Island Sweet Skunk, Ghost Train Haze, Chernobyl, ACDC, Amnesia, Sour Kush, Moby Dick, UK Cheese, SFV OG, Acapulco Gold, Purple Diesel, Pineapple, Grapefruit, Jack Frost, Super Sour Diesel, Casey Jones, Great White Shark, Haze, Jack the Ripper, $100 OG,

Golden Pineapple, Jesus OG, Sour Tangie, Power Plant, and Jack Flash could be used.

- *To become productive*, strains such as Green Crack, Jack Herer, Durban Poison, Super Lemon Haze, Chocolope, Harlequin, CinexCandy Jack, Phantom Cookies, Super Jack, Red Congolese, Allen Wrench, Green Ribbon, Sour Jack, Dirty Girl Clementine, Mickey Kush, Red Headed Stranger, Arjan's Strawberry Haze, Purple Arrow, , Island Sweet Skunk, Chernobyl, ACDC, J1, Acapulco Gold Purple Diesel, Grapefruit, Jack the Ripper, Critical Jack, Blue Crack Pandora's Box Grapefruit Diesel, Willie Nelson, Lemon Thai, Euforia, Mother's Helper, Colombian Gold, Kilimanjaro, Lemon Jack, Sour Tangie, Kali Mist, Jet Fuel, Alice in Wonderland, Chocolate Thai, Galactic Jack, Cracker Jack, Lucid Dream, Sweet Diesel, Pineapple Thai, and Green Dragon.

- *To become motivated*, strains such as Cinex, Mt. Hood Magic, Wonka's Bubblicious, Duke Nukem, Blue Boy, Alice in Wonderland,

Montana Silvertip, Fortune Cookies, Willie Nelson, Chocolate Thai, Super Snow Dog, Green Goblin, Galactic Jack, Nordle, Jacky White, Euforia, MediHaze, Mother's Helper, Kilimanjaro, Lemon Jack, Ed Rosenthal Super Bud, Lemon J1, Snowcap, Cracker Jack, Sweet Cheese, Jamaican Dream, Pineapple Thai, Nordle, Jacky White, Euforia, MediHaze, Mother's Helper, Kilimanjaro, Lemon Jack, Afghani Bullrider, Red Congolese, Sour Jack 303 OG, Malawi, Caramelicious, Irene OG Swazi Gold, DelaHaze,, Lemon Alien Dawg, Caramel Candy Kush, Wreck, Pineapple OG, Kali Mist Candy Jack, Super Jack, Tutankhamon, Critical Jack, Canna-Tsu, Chocolope Kush, Lemon Thai, 8 Ball, Kushand Peaches and Cream could be used.

- *To induce sleep*, strains such as OG Kush, Romulan, Cannatonic, Kosher Kush, Lavender, Larry OG, Afgoo, Vanilla Kush, Afghani, Dr. Who, Hash Plant, Grape God, Strawberry Kush, Lemon OG Kush OG #18, Blueberry Haze, Yoda OG Black Domina, Bubba OG, Mendocino Purps, Diablo, Paris OG, Death

Bubba, King Louis XIII, Platinum Kush, Blue Cheese, Purple Kush, God's Gift, LA Confidential, Tahoe OG Kush, Purple Urkle, Mazar x Blueberry, Blueberry Kush Sensi Star, God Bud, Pink Kush, Blackberry, , Platinum Bubba Kush, Diamond OG, Purple OG Kush Jedi Kush, Bubblegum Kush, Ace of Spades, Plushberry, Pure Kush, Pre-98 Bubba Kush, Querkle, XXX OG Purple Candy, and Monster Cookies could be used.

- *For anxiety*, strains such as Banana Kush, Silver Haze, White Dawg, Bubblicious, Blue Satellite, Cindy White, Cat Piss, Pure Power Plant, Glass Slipper, Trinity, Sour Grape, Green Dream, Cherry Bomb, Champagne Kush, Huckleberry, White Walker Kush, Brainstorm Haze, Viper, Dream Beaver, Orange Crush, Stardawg, 707 Headband Power Plant, Dragon's Breath, Pineapple Diesel, Citrix, Pineapple Skunk, Early Girl, Kaboom, Super Lemon OG, Armageddon, Black Mamba, Timewreck, Maui, Killer Queen, Sour Cheese, Tangilope, Raskal OG, Arjan's Strawberry Haze, Blue Goo, Atomic Northern Lights,

Rainbow, White Buffalo, Sugar Shack, Hawaiian Haze, Super Green Crack, Neville's Haze, Double, Tangie Banana, Avi-Dekel, and Super Sweet could be used.

- *To treat migraines and headaches*, strains such as Blue Dream, Amnesia, J1, Ghost Train Haze, SAGE, Cat Piss, Blueberry Headband, Platinum GSC, Fire OG, Banana Kush, Jillybean, Candyland, Lemon Skunk, Lamb's Bread, Romulan, Jedi Kush, Red Dragon, Chemdawg 4, Power Plant, Cherry Kush, Sour Kush, Sweet Tooth, Khalifa Kush, Grapefruit, Kandy Kush, Herijuana, Deadhead OG, Mango, True OG, Platinum Bubba Kush, Purple OG Kush, Super Lemon Haze, Master Kush, Cherry Pie, Maui Wowie, Death Star, LA Confidential, Kryptonite, 3 Kings, Bubblegum Kush, Pure Kush, Rockstar, Sour Diesel, Green Crack, Pineapple Express, Trainwreck, Nebula, Pure Power Plant, Vortex, and Cannalope Haze could be used.

- *To manage depression*, strains such as OG Kush, Obama Kush, Afgoo, King Louis XIII,

ACDC, Platinum Kush, Sensi Star, Flo, God Bud, Sweet Tooth, Pink Kush AK-47, Headband, Blue Cheese, Purple Kush, Chemdawg, God's Gift, Banana Kush, XJ-13, Lamb's Bread, White Fire OG, Cannatonic, Kosher Kush, Bubble Gum, Blueberry Kush, Grapefruit, Kandy Kush, Lavender, Larry OG, , Blackberry, Blue Diesel, UK Cheese, White Russian, Acapulco Gold, Purple Diesel, Pineapple, LA Confidential, Tahoe OG Kush, Platinum GSC Purple Urkle, Mazar x Blueberry, Golden Goat, Mango Kush, Berry White, Purple Haze, Bruce Banner, Fire OG, Pre-98 Bubba Kush, Vanilla Kush, and Super Sour Diesel could be used.

- *To treat arthritis*, strain such as Harlequin, Swazi Gold, Cheesewreck, Hawaiian Dream, Hellfire OG, Grape God, Afgooey, Pennywise, Tora Bora, CBD Critical Cure, GG5, 501st OG, Sour Amnesia,The Truth, Purple Voodoo, Ambrosia, CBD Shark, Bordello, Grapefruit Diesel, Lemon Thai, Purple Gorilla, Master Bubba, Zombie OG, Y Griega Warlock, Double Dream, Blueberry Haze, Harle-Tsu, Jet Fuel,

Ice, Cookies Kush, Tangerine Kush, Charlotte's Web, Tangerine, Cataract Kush, Master Yoda, Hell's OG, Grape Kush, Lemon G, Canna-Tsu, Scooby Snacks, Pandora's Box, Cannatonic, Critical Mass, ACDC, Flo, Afghani, , Medibud, Hardcore OG, and Sunshine Daydream could be used.

- *To fight off stomach ache and cramps*, strains such as Cheese Quake, Purple Mr. Nice, Green Crack Extreme, Rockstar Kush, Skunk Haze, Blue Champagne, Sour Haze, Afghan Haze, Sour Pebbles, Critical Widow, Blue Velvet, Zen, Digweed, Funky Monkey, Sputnik, Medicine Woman, Double OG, Aliens on Moonshine, Moloka'i Frost, Fat Purple, Double Barrel OG, Crystalberry, and Taliban Poison could be used.

- *To deal with stress*, strains such as AK-47, Headband, Purple Urkle, Golden Goat, Mango Kush, Bruce Banner, Fire OG, Banana Kush, Romulan, Cannatonic, Blue Cheese, ACDC, Flo, Sweet Tooth, Pink Kush, Blue Diesel, Acapulco Gold, Blue Magoo, Platinum Bubba Kush,

Purple OG Kush, Black Jack, Ogre, Bubblegum Kush, Ace of Spades, OG #18, Yoda OG, Harle-Tsu, Jet Fuel, Pineapple Chunk, Strawberry Diesel, Diablo, DJ Short Blueberry, Purple Diesel, Pineapple, Kandy Kush, Pre-98 Bubba Kush, Vanilla Kush, Super Sour Diesel, Great White Shark, Golden Pineapple, Permafrost, Chemdawg, Platinum GSC, Kosher Kush, Lemon OG Kush, Querkle, Key Lime Pie, Dogwalker OG, Mango Haze, and Redwood Kush could be used.

- *To find relief from epileptic seizure*, strains such as Big Bang, Frosted Freak, Romulan Grapefruit, Lemon Pie, Frisian Dew, Alohaberry, Argyle, black Bubba, TJ's CBD, Dreamer's Glass, Devil Fruit, Brandywine, Maui Haole, Marcosus Marshmellow, GI001, Darkside OG, Gorilla Biscuit, Southern Lights, Athabasca, G.O.A.T., Blackberry Dream, Bedford Glue, Redd Cross, Bell Ringer, and F'n LouZER could be used.

- *For the treatment of inflammatory disorders*, strains such as Harlequin, Cannatonic, Critical

Mass, Obama Kush, ACDC, Flo, Afghani, Grape God, Blue Widow, Afgooey, Blueberry Headband, Pennywise, 707 Headband, Double Dream, Blueberry Diesel, OG #18, Blueberry Haze, Harle-Tsu, Jet Fuel, Blue Haze, Ice, Quantum Kush, Cookies Kush, Tangerine Kush, Charlotte's Web, Sour Tsunami, Tangerine, Shark Shock, Super Jack, Cataract Kush, Master Yoda, Northern Lights #5, Dirty Girl, Hell's OG, Cherry Bomb, Grape Kush, Chemdawg 91, Lemon G, Canna-Tsu, Scooby Snacks, Ingrid, Pandora's Box, Snoop Dogg OG, Grapefruit Diesel, Alien Kush, Confidential Cheese, Lemon Thai, and Purple Gorilla could be used.

- *To help reduce fatigue*, strain such as Green Crack, Jet Fuel, Super Jack, Purple Diesel, Duke Nukem, Jack Herer, Durban Poison, Super Lemon Haze, Red Congolese, Allen Wrench, Sour Jack, Dirty Girl, Clementine, Critical Jack, Blue Crack, Grapefruit Diesel, Willie Nelson, Mother's Helper, Kilimanjaro, Mickey Kush, Red Headed Stranger, Island Sweet Skunk, Chernobyl, Acapulco Gold,

Strawberry Ice, Alice in Wonderland, Chocolate Thai, Lucid Dream, Malawi, Jack's Cleaner, DelaHaze, Y Griega, Blue Trainwreck, Chocolope, Harlequin, Cinex, Seattle Cough, Pink Lemonade, Mexican Sativa, Moose and Lobsta, White Siberian, Grapefruit, Jack the Ripper, Sour Tangie, Kali Mist, Arjan's Strawberry Haze, Aloha, Shaman, Purple Jack, and Blue Dot could be used.

PRECAUTIONS FOR USING STRAINS

It should be noted that most of the strains that have been mentioned above have a high THC content and will cause psychoactive effects. The strains that could help with several of these issues and other disorders have been mention in detail before this section; they have a high Cannabidiol (CBD) percentage. The higher CBD percentage allows the strains to work better as it has no psychoactive effects and all the benefits. Tetrahydrocannabinol (THC) cannabinoid is one of the main constituents of most strains as they are bred for merely recreational purposes. However,

THC does have some beneficial properties, but they are weighed down by the side effects caused by this cannabinoid.

Long-term use of THC high strain could cause many adverse effects on the body. It could cause anxiety, paranoia, hallucinations, panic, loss of sensation, increased heart rate, coordination impairment, and many other problems through the short-term use of THC high strains. Other adverse effects that could originate in THC high strain users are mood swings, poor academic performance, addiction, opiate addiction, sexual problems, antisocial behavior, behavioral issues, and many other similar issues.

Strains that have a 1:1 ratio or an equal ratio of CBD and THC cannabinoid should only be used when the individual is suffering from severe disorders that could not be dealt with the standard measures of medicine. Individuals that have mild to moderate disorders should choose a strain that has a very low THC ratio and a higher CBD ratio as they would be more beneficial and quicker in dealing with the issues.

Patients that need to begin using a strain for their disorders or diseases should first consult their doctors, as some strains may irritate the conditions due to the presence of THC cannabinoid. For example, THC high strain could cause patients suffering from migraine have momentary relief, but when the effects wear off adverse effects such as headaches and irritated eyes might become a problem.

Those who suffer from very mild mental health issues such as general anxiety should not opt for the use of these strain, hey can get better mental health by adding CBD hemp oil supplements into the diet. As the general CBD hemp oil has anxiolytic properties that could help them find relief from anxiety-related disorders. It is recommended to use strains of CBD when the individual has a disorder or a disease that hinders the daily life of the individual such as epileptic seizures, severe chronic pain, severe PTSD, chronic inflammatory disorders, and so forth.

CHAPTER SIX - A BRIEF GUIDE TO A HEALTHIER LIFE

Changing the routine lifestyle style could be hard, most of us opt to live the easier path that only helps us for a short time. Our rational mind does not always bring us to better results, in the end, rather it tries to bring quicker and efficient results. Sometimes, it is necessary to think outside the box to set a proper and healthier long-term goal. By incorporating a few habits into your lives, we can see a lot of change in our lifestyles and health. This chapter is dedicated to providing a better and healthier routine by suggesting easier and quicker habits. By adopting these habits into the lifestyle, one could have better health, skin, and higher energy levels.

JUMP ON TO THE NUTRITION BANDWAGON

Eating is one of the most important parts of our daily lives if we eat properly then many of our issues could not be dealt with any medicine. The motivation to eat is ruined if the food is unhealthy, which is why it is important to find healthier and tastier alternative to the necessary nutrients in our body. There are several nutrients that can become a proper source of healing if they are taken in the right way.

INTAKE OF IRON

Iron is an essential nutrient that needs by men and women; it is responsible for the growth and health of our nervous system. Our body needs a better quality of iron rather than the quantity, which is why it is better to eat better than in larger amounts. It is a good thing that iron is available in many vegetables and plants, where the quality of Iron has the best consistency.

Iron is readily available in red meat that can be easily added to the lunchtime meal by adding it to a salad or a sandwich. Baked beans and peas are also a great source of iron, which can be incorporated as a side meal at dinner times. Other vegetables that are abundant in iron are cabbages, kidney beans, tomatoes, spinach, and broccoli.

INTAKE OF PROTEIN

Protein is responsible for the healthier growth of our hair, skins, and nails. This mineral also helps the production of hormones and enzymes that could potentially repair cartilage, muscles, bones, bones, and skin. The addition of this nutrient is very important; it can be easily added to the diet by addition of healthier alternatives. Hemp seed oil has an abundance of protein; it could be added to smoothies to make it healthier and tastier version.

Legumes, nuts, and beans are also a great source of inexpensive protein. You can cook a batch of black beans and hummus and use them regularly for your meals. It is a quick and easy way to boost the health meter up on a busy day. Protein snacks could easily be made through high protein ingredients such as yogurt, eggs, cheeses, and low-fat milk. A tablespoon of hemp seed has approximately 10 grams of protein so it could be a great addition by adding it into your daily routine.

INTAKE OF HEALTHIER FATS AND OILS

Many oils that are commonly used in our daily lives are processed and can cause the individual to have higher cholesterol levels. Some oils have saturated fats that are harmful to the body, while other have saturated fats that can help the body to become stronger. Saturated fats can increase the risk of a stroke and heart attack, which is why it is important that the amount of saturated fat in the daily diet is less than 10%.

 There are some oils that are heat processed and have several chemical solvents that make them unhealthy for our diet. Some of the oils that should be avoided are canola oil, peanut oil, sunflower oil, corn oil, grapeseed oil, margarine, safflower oil, cottonseed oil, shortening, soybean oil, "vegetable" oil and any other fake butter substitutes.

Healthier alternatives to this oil are coconut oil that has lauric acid; hemp seed oil can be added in little amounts into coconut oil to prepare various snacks. Even butter is a healthier alternative as it has K2,

Vitamin A, E, also many other elements that help in improving the health. Palm oil, olive oil, and avocado oil can be used for cooking as they are filled with vitamins and other nutrients.

HEALTHIER INGREDIENT CHOICES

Many ingredients that we choose to add in our food are processed, which makes them lose their nutrient content and become unhealthy. The processed food contains a lot of chemicals that could cause more harm to the body than healing. Here are some food choices that should be avoided and alternatives that could be used.

- Most of us know that eating sugar in high amounts can cause devastating effects on the metabolism and it will make the calorie count go hay-wire. Sugar and fructose corn syrup is the main cause of strokes, diabetes, and cancer. A better alternative to sugar is natural sweeteners such as Molasses, agave nectar, sucanat, and maple syrup.

- Refined grains that have been processed at least once have all the good stuff removed, so it is better to avoid them. Instead of using refined grained, it better to use whole grains.

Many seeds are loaded with protein, healthy fats, minerals, vitamins, proteins, dietary fiber, and anti-oxidants. There are many types of seeds that you can add to your meals which can boost the flavor and crunch of a meal.

- Hemp seeds are very common to find at the grocery store; they are getting increasingly popular in food stores with dressings, desserts, and chips. These seeds are very easy to eat as they soft; they are also a source of protein, all essential amino acids, and fatty acids. You can eat them by adding them to your cereal or baked goods. You can also add these to your smoothies, sprinkle them on your meals like pasta or stews.

- Pumpkin seed can also be used for medicinal purposes as they have potent anti-inflammatory abilities. They could be added to the cereal or eaten as a snack by themselves.

- Sunflower seed has many constituents such as folate, iron, protein, dietary fiber, zinc, and vitamin E. These seeds can help the body by preventing cardiovascular diseases. It is also a mild anti-oxidant that could be used to get rid of bad cholesterol levels.

- Sesame seeds are commonly used on bread and buns as they have a great taste. However, this seed is a great source of iron, magnesium, zinc, phosphorus, dietary fiber, and vitamins. This seed also has anti-inflammatory properties that could improve the overall health. These could be added to a salad or sprinkled on steamed veggies to make it tastier and healthier.

Process flour has a very few vitamins and natural minerals. The good qualities of flour stripped away during processing to make it look cleaner. This type of white flour that is processed for its looks rather than quality can cause high blood pressure, obesity, fatty liver disease, diabetes, increased risk of inflammatory disease and cancer; it can also cause anxiety and low energy levels.

There are several healthier alternatives to white flour such as whole wheat flour that is the unprocessed and healthier version of white flour. Spelt flour is also a great alternative as it has a high amount of protein. Brown rice flour that has a distinct nutty flavor can also be added into other healthier flours for additional taste. Millet flour is another great alternative as it is filled with vitamins and minerals, it has a creamy flavor and can be added to other flour. Soy flour is a great source of nutrients as it is high in protein. Rye flour can also be used to make bread and snacks as it is jam-packed with flavor and taste. Hemp flour that is made by crushing dried hemp seeds is also a very good alternative to white flour as it has proteins and unsaturated fats that could be beneficial for the body.

Seasonings are also a great source of nutrition as they have become an important part of our diet. Like many other food items, some seasonings are better than the commonly used seasonings. Sage is a healthy herb that could be used to treat a sore throat and boost the memory. It can be mixed with parsley, squashes, walnuts, thyme, and rosemary. Herbalist has also confirmed that sage can help individuals suffering from Alzheimer's.

Rosemary has mild anti-bacterial abilities that could kill the bad bacteria present in the food. It can be paired with potatoes, garlic, honey, citrus, peppers, and onions to present a tasty dish. Rosemary is used in aromatherapy because it has properties that could heighten mental focus, it is a mild anti-oxidant as well. Turmeric is a natural anti-inflammatory herb; it can also inhibit the growth of tumors in the body. It can be paired with curry, coriander, cumin, and garlic.

Chile peppers can help boost metabolism and can naturally lower the temperature of our bodies. It can be paired with bean, ginger, and beef. Ginger is a natural anti-inflammatory and can help patients that struggle with arthritis find relief. It can be used to soothe stomach ache and other issues. It can be paired with citrus, soy sauce, and garlic.

Cinnamon can also be used to stabilize blood sugar levels that can be paired with cloves, allspice, nutmeg, and nuts. Saffron can be used by individuals that have mood disorders to stabilize moods; it is also known to relieve the symptoms of PMS. It can be paired with rice, garlic, onion, and shellfish. Parsley is known to inhibit the growth of cancer cells; it can be paired with mint, lemon zest, capers, garlic, beef and fish in many dishes.

Oregano is a natural anti-bacterial that could fight against the bad bacteria present in our bodies. It can be paired with spinach, olive oil and vinegar to make a tasty dish. Nutmeg can be used as an antibacterial to prevent many issues; it can be paired with coffee, chickpeas, and cinnamon.

By using these healthier alternatives, one can maintain a healthier body and increase the productivity rate. Unhealthy foods lower the productivity rate of the body by hindering many of the natural processes of the body. When the body has a healthy and proper diet, it can work efficiently. By using the healthier alternatives, irregular mood and behavior could also be maintained as it can boost the mood by offering an energetic body. Healthier eating can also improve the longevity of individuals, regardless if they are suffering from disorders or diseases.

THE 5-A-DAY RULE

This campaign started as a method to help people find a balanced diet with color coordinated food items. This does not mean that one has to eat five times a day to get a balanced diet, rather, it means there should be five portions in your meal including fruit, vegetables, meat, dairy, and other nutritional food items.

Many things can count as one portion of the five in your meal such as fresh cut up fruit or vegetables, some dried fruits as snacks, fruit juice or smoothies, and beans or pulses. It is recommended that the daily diet is divided into color groups for easier handling and division of portions.

Unsweetened fruit juice, fresh fruits with oatmeal or cereal, banana with any kind of whole grain bread, any kind of fruit smoothie with skimmed milk can count as a healthy breakfast according to 5-A-Day rule. Carrots batons, raisins, dried apricots, grapes, baby sweet corn, celery sticks enjoy these with a low-calorie dip can count as a healthy snack according to 5-A-Day rule.

Minced cucumber, tomato and onion salad with a good spicy dressing, vegetable chowder or soup is a very good choice as a healthy lunch. Whereas, boiled veggies, stir-fry veggies or fruit salad as a side dish with meat meal can count as a hale and hearty dinner proportion.

FOLLOW A SET EXERCISE ROUTINE

To keep a healthy body, one must exercise daily to keep the muscles and the bones strong. Most people find it incredibly boring and a waste of time, however, committing to this small practice could help them in the long run. One of the most important things to notice is that the quantity of the exercise does not matter, the quality does. It will not help the body if is taking breaks or using the phone every other minute in a half an hour routine.

INCORPORATING SUPPLEMENTS WITH THE WORKOUT

A proper exercise needs attention and quality time, which in turn will help the body become stronger. A good exercise routine has strength exercises and cardiovascular exercises, so it is important to switch between the two during a short exercise regimen. It is also important to note that supplements such as hemp seed oils should be taken before the exercise routine. The exercise routine should be followed by a nutritional smoothie or juice with greens or healthy fruit to give your muscles energy for the rest of the day.

SIMPLE HOME WORKOUTS

A home exercise routine can be a great way to start the day; it does not need to take longer than 15 to 30 minutes. In the initial stages of the exercise routine, one should begin with smaller intensity sessions and move up as they feel more confident in moving their body. Exercises such as pushups, crunches, and jogging are one of the best beginner workouts to start from.

- **Jog:** To warm up the body, begin with jogging for around 15 to 20 minute and gradually increase the time as necessary.

- **Push-ups:** Once the body has warmed up, start by practicing 5 to 10 push-ups. It is important the push-up has a proper stance, and the elbows are not bent. It is better to do a smaller amount of complete push-ups rather than the fake push-ups that go halfway. A proper push up has the back straight and the head up, this exercises many muscles of the boy. Whereas, the fake push-ups only give the appearance of a push-up, without any benefits. Once, the routine has settled down start by gradually increasing the number of push-ups to 20 and so forth.

- **Crunches:** This exercise is an important part of the workout routine as it gives you a flatter stomach. They can help reduce the risk of osteoporosis, degenerative disc disease, back pain, and many other issues. A proper crunch has the elbows touching the knees at a controlled pace.

Hastening the pace of crunches does more damage, it could cause the muscle to cramp and ache all day. It is important to complete the crunches as you engage the back in a slow and controlled pace. Start with five crunches a day and increase the amount as the body becomes at-ease with regular workout.

RELAX YOUR MIND

It is important for our mind to relax and find peace everyone in a while so that it maintains a balanced and happy state. The constant stress of our daily lives could potentially cause our body to respond in worse ways. The relationship between relaxation and happiness is very complex, which in turn keeps our mental health balanced and maintained. It could affect our behaviors, emotions, energy, appetite, and relations. It could even be said that a healthy mind can make or break a worthwhile life. Relaxation can help our mind by setting a schedule and following it.

Preparing a schedule can help to maintain the division of your time during a busy schedule. So take out your pen and paper. Write down your work hours and free hours. Divide your work hours into actually working and working out during the intervals. Divide the free time at home to into working out, giving yourself time, and preparing a healthy meal for dinner and the next day. Stick to this schedule, don't worry if you don't completely and accurately follow it. Just try to slowly accumulate your life into a planned schedule, it will reduce stress considerably.

FIND A CALMER STATE OF MIND

Finding peace of mind is an important way for a healthy body. It is proven that by meditation, we can have a feeling of relaxation, lower blood pressure, less perspiration, and less stress. It can also deal with the release of the negative emotions that are built up in our mind. Through meditation, we can find a way to release the useless attachments to material things and a feeling of liberation from the things that are not under our control like external environment and circumstances. You can relax after a stressful day by taking a warm bath.

A mild CBD hemp oil drop to relax can also be used after a stressful day at work. It can be followed by meditation that can cleanse the mind as it is a great stress reliever and when you feel lesser stress it is easier to fall asleep. Some of the meditation technique that could be used to relax are concentration meditation and mindfulness meditation, both of which are the two most important and easiest meditation techniques that can set our mind on a healthier path. The basics of most meditation technique are as follows:

Sit down on the floor or grass, wherever is comfortable and close your eyes.

- Do not take control of your breathing, just let your body relax.

- Focus on how your body moves while you breathe, how your chest moves, and where the air completely dissolves in your body.

- If your mind wanders, bring the focus back to your body. Continue this technique for 4-5 minutes, increase the time as you get better.

CHAPTER SEVEN - HEALTHY CBD HEMP OIL/ HEMP OIL/ HEMP SEED RECIPES.

Before delving into the realm of recipes, let's learn about hemp oil as cooking oil. Hemp oil is considered to be a great alternative to fish oil that is why vegans often use it. It is very low in saturated fats that make it healthier than many other cooking oils. Hemp oil has a very dark color that has a green and yellow tint. It has to be refrigerated, or it will go rancid and lose its effectiveness.

It is best to use hemp oil that has been cold pressed from organic and non-GMO plants. The taste of hemp oil and seeds have an earthy and nutty flavor that can be used to make bread dips or dressings. It has a strong flavor which is why it is not often used in any sweet or delicate.

Hemp oil and CBD hemp oil have a very low smoke point, it will start to smoke when it is heated even a tiny bit. It cannot be used to deep fry or stir-fry because it cannot be heated, it can be warmed using warm water. However, this oil is perfect for salads and dips; it can also be used in pesto and hummus to give a tasty kick. Hemp oil can also be added to a smoothie in little amounts to make a tasty and healthy drink.

VEGAN HEMP SEED PESTO

This tasty pesto gives a delightful kick through a combination of nutty and earthy flavor that goes perfectly with fresh basils.

INGREDIENTS

Fresh basil   2 1/2 cups

Shelled hemp seeds   1/4 cup

Walnuts (or pine nuts)   1/4 cup

Fresh spinach   1 cup

Lemon (or lime juice)   1 tbsp.

Flax oil   1/4 cup

Olive oil (or hemp oil)   2 tbsp.

Garlic   3 cloves

Fresh ground black pepper and salt (to taste)

DIRECTION

1. First, coarsely chop basil and the spinach/parsley and put them in the blender, add the lemon juice and the hemp seeds into the blender as well. Give the mixture a few pulses in the blender.

2. Add olive oil and the flax oil into the mixture as it blends. Keep on blending the mixture until everything is properly combined.

3. To change the consistency to taste, a few drops of the oils can be added at this point.

4. Add fresh ground black pepper and salt into the mixture as taste. Enjoy as a dip or add into pasta to have a completely healthy and hearty meal.

RAW FOOD TRAIL MIX

Trail mixes are one of the healthy snacks that can be tweaked to taste and made into a nutritional combination. By taking a few extra steps and adding ingredients that can give you more health benefits, this trail mix can be made into something phenomenal.

INGREDIENTS

Walnuts   1 cup

Raw mulberries   1/2 cup

Deglet dates (pitted and diced)   1/2 cup

Hemp seeds   2 tablespoons

Dried fruit (such as chopped blueberries, pineapple, and cranberries)   1 cup

Cinnamon   1/2 teaspoon (optional)

Almonds   1 cup

Raw buckwheat groats, optional   1/2 cup

Goji berries   1/2 cup

Cardamom   1/2 teaspoon (Optional)

DIRECTIONS

1. Soak the buckwheat, almonds, and walnuts for over an hour. Drain and rinse all of them together. When dried, chop them into small pieces or chunks.

2. Next, spread the dried bits on a dehydrator tray and let them dry out at 145F for one to two hours. They should be crunchy and dry at this point. The chunks can also be dried out in the sun if the temperature is over 100F, it will take a few hours for them to become dry.

3. After drying them out, put the buckwheat, almonds, walnuts, and the rest of the ingredients in a zip-lock bag or a plastic bag. Combine the ingredients by shaking the mixture vigorously; all the spices should be evenly mixed.

4. The trail mix should be stored in an airtight container or jar that should be placed in the refrigerator or a cool room.

SUPERFOOD SALAD

This super salad is super simple to make and has some basics ingredients that can be up with other seasonal vegetables. It has a delightful mix of lemon, lentils, and hemp seeds that give this salad a boost in nutrients, making it worthwhile.

INGREDIENTS

Lentils (brown, black or green)   1 cup

Fine sea salt, plus more to taste   1 teaspoon

Garlic clove or shallot   1 small

Lemon   1

Freshly ground black pepper   1/4 teaspoon

Ground mustard   1/4 teaspoon

Extra virgin olive oil   3 Tablespoons

Green onions   1 to 5

Walnuts   to taste

Feta cheese (crumbled)   to taste

Fennel   to taste

Hemp seed   to taste

Toasted pine nuts   to taste

DIRECTIONS

1. First, the lentils have to be boiled in a large pot. Add six cups of water to the lentils and bring it to a boil. After it has boiled, lower the heat and let the water simmer. Check the lentils to see if they are half-way cooked, you can do that by checking the hardness of the lentils. Add salt to the simmering pot if the lentils are half-boiled and the center is half-way cooked. Simmer the lentils until they have become tender. Drain them and set aside for them to cool down.

2. In the meanwhile, let's make the dressing. Mince the peeled shallots/garlic and put them in a large bowl. Add one teaspoon of lemon zest to the bowl, be careful as to avoid adding the bitter part of the lemon into the bowl. Cute the lemon in half and squeeze its juice into the bowl. Add the mustard and pepper into the

concoction and mix it with a whisk. Leave it aside for five minutes and whisk in the olive oil.

3. Dry of the lentils and shake off any excess water on the lentils. Add the drained lentils into the bowl. Toss the lentils and the dressing until the lentils have been evenly coated by the dressing.

4. You can add toasted pines, fennel, feta cheese, and hemp seeds into the salad at this point. Simply, toss the salad so that the added ingredients have even coating of the dressing.

TABOULI SALAD

Tabouli Salad is jam-packed with several vegetables and herbs that are known as superfoods. This salad is made with parsley and cilantro, both which have properties to act as detoxifiers that can clean the toxins.

INGREDIENTS

Parsley   1 bunch (chopped)

Cilantro   1 bunch (chopped)

Green Onions   1 bunch (Sliced)

Agave or Honey (optional)   1 Tbsp.

Avocado   1(chopped)

Hemp Seeds or Almonds   ½ cup (coarsely ground)

Tomatoes   2chopped

Olive Oil   2 Tbsp.

Lemon   half (Juiced)

Salt   1 Tsp.

Cayenne   to taste

DIRECTIONS

1. First, wash the cilantro and parsley, cute off their stems and put them in the food processor. Process the cilantro and parsley until they are chopped into small pieces.

2. Dice the avocado, onions, and tomatoes into small cubes and put them in a bowl. Add the rest of the ingredients into the bowl as well.

3. Mix the chopped cilantro and parsley into the bowl and serve.

HEMP AND CARROT SOUP

This tasty delight will rouse your taste buds and give you a protein filled meal in a small amount of time.

INGREDIENTS

Hemp Oil   1/4 cup

Shelled hemp seed   3tbsp.

Carrots, chopped   4 cups

Water   3 cups

White onion   1/4 cup (chopped)

Parsley   1/4 cup

Arugula or spinach   1/4 cup

 Sun-dried tomato   1/4 cup

Dried oregano   1 tbsp.

Avocado   1 (chopped)

Lemon juice   1/4 cup

DIRECTIONS

1. Cut the carrots into smaller chunks and add them to the blender. Add the onions, parsley, spinach, tomatoes, oregano, and lemon juice into the blender as well. Add three cups of

water and blend all of the things in the blender until they are smooth and creamy.

2. Pour the creamy mixture into a pot and bring to a boil before serving them. Add the avocado and hemp seeds in the mixture before serving for a tasty kick.

SPICY CHICKPEAS AND CUCUMBER SALAD

What is a healthy snack list without a salad? This protein-packed meal is the best ready-made snack you can have in your fridge to eat any time you are peckish.

INGREDIENTS

Rice Vinegar	½ Cup
Natural Cane Sugar	1 ½ -2 Tbsp
Fine Grain Sea Salt	½ Tsp.
Hemp oil	½ Tsp

Cucumber	2
Red Pepper	1, Diced
Red Onion	1 Cup, Diced
Cilantro	¼ Cup, Chopped
Roasted Peanuts	¼ Cup, Chopped
Spiced Chickpeas	For Garnish

DIRECTIONS

1. Whisk the vinegar, cane sugar, hemp oil, and the salt in a small bowl. Adjust the sweet taste as you prefer. Set it aside. Peel the cucumber, half it length-wise. Take out the seeds and slice the halved so that they make a moon shape. Put them in a medium-size bowl. Dice the onion and red pepper into the bowl. Roughly dice the cilantro and add it to the bowl.

2. Pour the dressing into the bowl and toss the salad. Let the salad sit for 20 minutes in the fridge. In the meantime roast the chickpeas.

Toss them into the salad and serve immediately.

HEMP BURGERS

Ever need to fill the blank space left behind by junk food? Worry no more, hemp burgers offers a guilt-free pathway for people to enjoy a tasty meal.

INGREDIENTS

Soft tofu   10 ounces

Shelled hemp seeds   1 cup

Sunflower seeds   1/4 cup

Scallions   1/4 cup (chopped)

Soy sauce   2 Tbs.

Nutritional yeast   2 Tbs.

Dried basil   1/2 tsp.

Herb seasoned stuffing   2 cups

DIRECTIONS

1. First, puree the tofu in a blender. Add the shelled hemp seeds, sunflower seeds, chopped scallions, soy sauce, nutritional yeast, and dried basil into the puree and give it a blend.

2. Put the herb stuffing in a bowl and pour the tofu mixture on top. Mix both of the concoctions well and form patties.

3. Bake the patties on a greased cookie sheet for 25 to 30 minutes at about 300F. The patties should be golden brown at this point.

TOFU TACOS

Anything is better with tacos, am I right or am I right? Here is a tasty and satisfying breakfast that even those meat eaters can't resist.

INGREDIENTS

Whole wheat flour   ¼ cup

Yeast	¼ cup
Onion powder	2 tsp.
Garlic powder	½ tsp
Extra-firm tofu	14- ounce
Turmeric	¼ tsp.
Corn tortillas	8
Salsa	as preferred
Soy sauce	2 tbsp.

Toppings include: onion, greens, potato, avocado, shelled hemp seeds and cilantro   a handful

DIRECTIONS

1. First, we need to drain the tofu, put a heavy plate on it for 20-30 minutes. Crumble the dried tofu in a bowl and sprinkle it with flour, yeast, onion powder, garlic powder, and turmeric. Mix it while tossing, add the soy sauce in-between.

2. Heat a non-stick pan over medium heat, cook the tofu mixture and keep on stirring, so it doesn't stick to the pan. When the tofu turns brown and crisp, serve with warm tortillas. Add salsa and toppings as you prefer.

GRILLED TOMATO SALSA

This salsa is best served with tortilla crisps or crackers.

INGREDIENTS

Ripe Tomatoes   4 (Halved and Seeded)

Red Onions   ½ (Finely Chopped)

Red Chillies   2 Cloves (Seeded and Finely Chopped)

Fresh Coriander   A Handful(Chopped)

Olive Oil   1 Tbsp.

Lemon Juice   1 Tbsp.

Hemp oil   ½ tsp.

Black Pepper.   To Taste

DIRECTIONS

1. Turn on the grill, arrange the halved tomatoes on the baking tray. Grill them until they are darkened, it will take 5 minutes. Let them cool down for 20 minutes.

2. Remove the tomato skin, discard it. In a medium bowl place the tomatoes after chopping them. Add the garlic, red chilies, red onion, olive oil, hemp oil, coriander, lemon juice, pepper, and salt, mix it and let it sit for an hour before serving.

VEGAN MAC N CHEESE

This yummy goodness will give you a trip back to your childhood. It is the same but so different, this is wholesome, unprocessed, dairy-free goodness.

INGREDIENTS

Large Macaroni Shells / Pipe Rigate   10 Ounces

White Onions   ½ (Diced)

Garlic   3-4 Cloves

Minced, Raw Cashews   1 Cup (Soaked For 5-6 Hrs.)

Vegetable Broth   1 ½ Cups

Cornstarch   1 Tbsp.

Cumin   ½ Tsp.

Chili Powder   ¾ Tsp.

Nutritional Yeast   2 Tbsp.

Green Chili   14 Ounce, Diced

CBD hemp oil   1/2 tsp.

Tortilla Chips   1 Cup(Optional)

DIRECTIONS

1. Boil the macaroni according to the given instructions on the package. In the meantime, if you want the mac n cheese to be topped with

crunchy chips then crush the chips and place them on a baking sheet lined with parchment paper. Bake them for 10 minutes on 350 F; they will turn golden brown.

2. Sate the garlic and onion in a medium skillet with olive oil. Season it as you prefer with salt and pepper. Cook for 8 minutes and set it aside. Add the garlic and onion into a blender with the rest of the ingredients except the hemp oil, but only half of the chili and blend until smooth and creamy.

3. Drain the mac and let it dry. In the same pot with the drained water, add the cashew cream and stir on low heat until it slightly thickens. Add the mac and the hemp oil to the cheese and stir. Add the rest of the chilies and top it off with cilantro and tortilla chips. Serve while hot. It will make four servings.

CREAMY AVOCADO PASTA

This creamy delight is for all those avocado lovers out there. It's cooked with a creamy avocado paste with loads of garlic, tres been!

INGREDIENTS

Whole-Wheat Tagliatelle   170g

Lemon   ½ (Juiced And Zested)

Salt   ½ Tsp.

Olive Oil   2 Tbsp.

Hemp Oil   ½ Tsp.

Garlic Clove   2, Minced

Avocado   1, Pitted

Black Pepper   To Taste

DIRECTIONS

1. Boil the tagliatelle as instructed on the box, it usually takes 8-10 minutes. In another bowl, add salt, olive oil, lemon juice and the minced garlic and mince the avocado in it.

2. When the pasta is cooked, drain it and transfer it to another bowl. Pour the avocado sauce on it and toss it until it is completely covered. Garnish with black pepper and lemon zest. Serve while hot.

VEGAN CHILLI

Want to spice up your dinner? Then this chili with many fragrant spices will create the best hearty and healthy chili you ever had.

INGREDIENTS

Soya Mince	350g
Tin Kidney Beans	400g
Red Onion	1, Chopped
Celery Stalks	4, Diced
Red Pepper	2, Chopped
Bay Leaves	4 Bay Leaves
Chili Powder	2 Tbsp.

Treacle	3 Tbsp.
Stock Cube	1
Fresh Coriander	A Handful
Hot Sauce	1 Tsp.
Black Pepper	To Taste
Shelled Hemp seeds	To Taste
Water	3 Tbsp.
Plain Flour	225ml.

DIRECTIONS

1. Combine the kidney beans, celery, onions, red pepper, bay leaves, soy mince, chili powder, stock, treacle, coriander, hot sauce, salt and pepper in a slow cooker with 225ml water. Cook on high heat for 3 hrs.

2. Dissolve the flour in 225 hot water and pour it in the cooked chili. Let it cook for another hour. Serve by sprinkling it hemp seeds. It will make 8 servings.

PEANUT BUTTER GRANOLA

This is not a full blown breakfast, it can be a side dish to a good smoothie or even made for brunch.

INGREDIENTS

Peanut butter	2 tbsp.
Maple syrup or brown rice syrup	2 tbsp.
Cinnamon	¼ tsp.
Vanilla	¼ Tsp.
Oats	1 cup
Hemp seeds	to taste

DIRECTIONS

1. Heat the oven to 325 F. Spray a cookie sheet with non-stick cooking spray. Combine the peanut butter and syrup, mix until the peanut butter completely dissolves. It will take 20

seconds. Stir in the vanilla, oats, and cinnamon.

2. Spread out this mixture on the sheet and bake for 7-9 minutes. The granola will be slightly brown. Let it cool down and sprinkle with the hemp seeds. Eat it with a serving of sliced bananas, with a dash of maple syrup.

HIDDEN GREEN POWER SMOOTHIE

Looking to start the day with energy packed a tasty smoothie yet? Well here is your lucky day! This smoothie is vegan, gluten free, grain free, raw, sugar-free, and soy free.

INGREDIENTS

Unsweetened Almond Milk	1 ½ Cups
Organic Kale/ Baby Spinach	1 Cup
Large Medjool Dates (Optional)	1-2
Hulled Hemp Seed	3 Tbsp.
Unsweetened Cocoa Powder	2 Tbsp.

Frozen Banana	1
Cinnamon	A Dash
Avocado	1 Tbsp.
Ice (Optional)	½ Cup

DIRECTIONS

1. Make sure the dates are pitted. Add all the ingredients into a blender and blend until it shows a smooth consistency. Serve chilled.

GREEN WARRIOR PROTEIN SMOOTHIE

This is a great cool down creamy, cold, and luxurious smoothie for those hot summer mornings. Talk about a supercharged meal in a glass!

INGREDIENTS

| Red Grapefruit Juice | ½ Cup |
| Dinosaur/ Lacinato Kale | 1 Cup |

Apple	1, Cored And Roughly Chopped.
Cucumber	1 Cup
Celery	½ Cup
Shelled Hemp Seeds	3-4 Tbsp.
Mango	¼ Cup
Mint Leaves	1/8 Cup
Virgin Coconut Oil	½ Tbsp.
Ice Cubes	3-4 Ice Cubes.

DIRECTIONS

Add all the ingredients in a blender and blend until smooth consistency, add a dash of water if the mixture is thick. It will make two servings easily. Serve chilled.

FRUIT KABOBS

These kabobs have the creamiest dressing ever, raw cashews for the base of this cream. Drizzle it on the fruits and enjoy a nutrient snack.

INGREDIENTS

Raw Cashews   1 Cup

Almond Milk Or Any Non-Dairy Milk   ½ Cup + 1-2 Tbsp.

Cherries ½ Cup

Vanilla Extract   1 Tsp.

CBD hemp oil   2-3 drops

Coconut Nectar Syrup Or Liquid Sweetener Of Choice 2-3 Tbsp.

Fruit Of Choice: Strawberries, Cantaloupe, Grapes, Nectarines, Kiwi, Watermelon Etc. A Bowlful

DIRECTIONS

- Put cashews and water covering the nuts in a bowl, soak it overnight. Add almond milk, drained cashews, pitted cherries, vanilla, CBD hemp oil and sweetener in a blender. Blend the mixture until smooth consistency, add more milk if it thick and grainy. Chill this mixture or enjoy at room temperature.

- Make fruit cubes, skewer them, and drizzle them with this cream. Enjoy.

CHOCOLATE ALMOND FROZEN BANANA POPS

This dessert is as easier as it gets! Both adults and kids will surely love this banana recipe.

The ingredients are enough to make 4 servings

INGREDIENTS

Bananas   4

Almond butter	1/2cups
Vanilla extract	1/2tsp.
Cinnamon	1/4tsp.
Dark chocolate chunks	12 z.
CBD infused coconut oil	2 tbsp.
Popsicle sticks	4 wooden Popsicle sticks

DIRECTIONS

2. Place a banana on each of the Popsicle sticks.

3. Mix the vanilla, almond butter, and cinnamon.

4. On the curve of each banana, spread two tbsp. of the almond butter.

5. Melt the chocolate in a small bowl with the microwave and add the CBD-infused coconut oil in the melted chocolate. Pour the chocolate mixture into a tall glass. Dip the bananas in this mixture and place them on parchment paper placed on a plate.

6. Put them in the refrigerator until the chocolate is firm and serve

BANANA CREAM PIE BLIZZARDS

This creamy dessert will be an all-star at all your dinner dessert talks.

INGREDIENTS

Raw Cashews   1 Cup (Soaked For 6 Hours Or Overnight)

Unsweetened Almond Milk Or Coconut Milk   1 Cup

Vanilla Extract   1 Tsp.

Medjool Dates   5-7, Pitted

Banana Powder   2 Tbsp.

CBD-infused Coconut Oil   2 Tbsp.

Ripe Banana   1, Sliced

Vegan-Friendly Cookies (Optional)   A Handful (Crushed)

DIRECTIONS

1. Freeze the canister for 24 hours in which you will freeze this ice-cream and soak the cashew beforehand. Grind the banana chips in a coffee grinder or a spice grinder. Some parts won't grind take them out and save them for later.

2. Blend all the ingredients except raw banana and cookies until it turns creamy and smooth. Add more banana powder or dates to your taste. Chill this banana mixture for 2 hrs. or overnight if you don't have an ice cream maker. Otherwise just churn the mixture in an ice cream mixture for 45 minutes.

3. Scoop the ice cream out if firm then serves with crushed cookies, otherwise freeze if it for 2 hours.

CONCLUSION

Adding the CBD Hemp oil and its derivatives to the daily regiment could be a challenge. However, this challenge can offer discoveries that can make a healthier and happier you. This book was made to provide you with a detailed overview of the benefits of CBD. We hope that this book has helped you discover an entirely new world. We hope we have helped you find out a newer and healthy side of hemp oil and CBD.

This will provide you with all the essential boosts you need in your life to make it healthier despite the mystical myths that shed a negative image of the properties of the Hemp plant. We hope this book has provided you with enough knowledge about Hemp and the various, uncountable effects it has on your inner and outer well-being.

Through this book, individuals that struggle with various disorders can find an easier lifestyle by understanding the roots of Hemp and CBD. By understanding the different types of CBD components, it should be easier for beginners to scope out the best herbal alternative. As many patients struggling with various disorders have no remedy, many have started to turn to the miraculous healing powers of Hemp and its cannabinoid components. Without the proper knowledge of these components, they may find themselves in deeper waters.

It should also be noted that where hemp oil has no arbitrary effects other than it being a nutritional oil, CBD hemp oil may have other properties. These properties are associated with the cannabinoid content present in its constituents. It may cause the individual to feel analgesic, an-inflammatory, and many other associated effects.

Misuse of CBD derivatives can cause the individuals to have mild side effect as it has potent active properties. It may cause a headache or an unfamiliar taste on the palate in the beginning. It is important to start slow and small with CBD products and gradually increase the amount as necessary.

Patients with severe ailments should be very cautious of CBD or other cannabinoid products as they may cause them to react. This book has given the basic guidelines for beginners that need to know the use of

CBD products. However, it does not provide a cemented path that the individual must follow to find relief. Each person has a different constitution, which is why they should find their own favorites herbs or products that could help them with their issues. The CBD benefits in this book have been described to help individuals understand the history, properties, and use of CBD and hemp products that may help them find a healthier and stable life.

REFERENCES

1. Mikuriya TH. *Marijuana in medicine: past, present, and future.* Calif Med. 1969;110(1):34-40.

2. Aldrich M. *History of therapeutic cannabis.* In: Mathre ML, eds. Cannabis in medical practice. Jefferson, NC: Mc Farland; 1997. p. 35-55.

3. Pinho AR. *Social and medical aspects of the use of cannabis in Brazil.* In: Rubin V, eds. *Cannabis and culture.* Paris: Mounton Publishers; 1975. p. 293-302.

4. Moreau JJ. Du Hachisch et de l'Alienation Mentale: Etudes Psychologiques. Paris: Librarie de Fortin Mason; 1845 (English edition: New York, Raven Press; 1972).

5. Gaoni Y, Mechoulam RJ. *Isolation structure and partial synthesis of an active constituent of hashish.* J Am Chem Soc. 1964;86:1646-7.

6. Carlini EA. *The good and bad effects of (-) trans-delta-9- tetrahydrocannabinol (D9-THC) on humans.* Toxicon. 2004;44(4):461-7.

7. Bab, I, et al. *"Cannabinoids and the Skeleton: from Marijuana to Reversal of Bone Loss."* Advances in Pediatrics., U.S. National Library of Medicine, www.ncbi.nlm.nih.gov/pubmed/19634029.

8. Price, Matt. *"Understanding The Differences Between Hemp and Cannabis."* Health Benefits of Medical Marijuana - Cannabis 101, Medical Jane, 13 July 2017, www.medicaljane.com/2015/01/14/the-differences-between-hemp-and-cannabis/.

www.ingramcontent.com/pod-product-compliance
Lightning Source LLC
Chambersburg PA
CBHW072258260726
48658CB00004BA/1101